# STEADFAST

## A Breast Cancer Survivor's Healing Journey that Bares All with a Message of Hope, Faith, Wisdom, and Love

1 Corinthians 15:58
"Therefore, my beloved brethren, be ye steadfast, unmoveable, always abounding in the work of the Lord, forasmuch as ye know that your labour is not in vain in the Lord."

## SHARON REJISTRE

ISBN 978-1-0980-6682-6 (paperback)
ISBN 978-1-0980-6683-3 (digital)

Christian Faith Publishing, Inc.
832 Park Avenue
Meadville, PA 16335
www.christianfaithpublishing.com

Printed in the United States of America

To
Dr. Alexander Rejistre Sr.,
Alexander Rejistre Jr.,
Aaron Rejistre,
and
Anais Rejistre
All of you were my reason to never give up. The reason I am able
to stand is knowing I am able to do life with you. Thank you for
being the real soldiers in this journey with me. Stay steadfast in
all that you do. Live. Love. Learn. Laugh. Let go and look up!

# CONTENTS

# ACKNOWLEDGMENT

I OWE ALL THANKS AND praise to my Savior, Jesus Christ. I owe Him all of me, and I intend on expressing that all of my days. I am a recipient of His wondrous grace, and to share this story with you is simply amazing. I know if I had not gone through this process, perhaps I would be a very different woman. I am so blessed to have had so many people in my life to thank, that if I tried to thank them, I am not sure I could remember them all.

But to the two people who are responsible for my being, my parents, Lois and Willie Hudson, I love you so much, and you know how I feel about all that you have done and still do for me and my awesome four! When I grow up, I am going to make you proud one of these days.

My sister, Robbin, and my brother, Willie, who neither of them ever complained at all the days and nights I needed help or wanted a freebie (no kid day), y'all are the best. I am honored to be your sister. I needed all those laughs!

Of course, all of my friends (who are really my family). I will not get in trouble; but I must list the best of them all, Targie Crumpton (I love you, sis), who came to my house one morning before the sun came up and cooked breakfast for us just because she loves us and enjoys the bragging right of cooking better grits than me (this back story is hilarious).

My three church families, Mt. Moriah MBC of Dumas, Arkansas, Marzell MBC of Gould, Arkansas, and Canaan Christian Center of Pine Bluff, Arkansas, these were some fasting and praying people! I thank you from the bottom of my heart. You all did so much, the whole congregation of three different churches. How rare is that? I cannot begin to mention everything you did, but you know what happened. And I need you to know I never forgot. I will not mention all by name, but the pastors of these churches were my lifeline. Pastor Johnny Morton and Lady Iris Morton, I love you and all that you have done for me and how you rallied the troops to frontlines for prayer, the love gifts, phone calls, and all that everyone did. Apostle Banks and Dr. Sheryl Banks, you truly went beyond the call of duty, and I will be grateful always for that. I salute you for being there for us and keeping it 1000, like they do in the land of big grapes! Pastor Lamar Brooks a.k.a. Uncle Mark and Auntie Bobbie you were there not only for me but the family as well. I love you and will forever be your favorite niece. I am made better for the anointing on our life keep on bringing the storm for Jesus.

I have to make mention of a few ladies in particular: Dr. Joanna Edwards, Dr. Josetta Wilkins (pink battle buddy), Christine Grandy (pink battle buddy), Flora Simon, Cheryl Townsend, Jonell Smith, Shenetta Jimmerson, Elaine Green (I owe you some major hair products and a few racks), Rosalyn Burks, Deborah Fisher (pink battle buddy), the ladies of BAD (Blessed and Delivered), you women were bad to the bone, and I am forever grateful for the commitment to stand with me. I will not mention you, but you know who you are.

And to my entire medical team, I prayed so much for you all and became like family with some. You were all so kind and patient with me. Again, how rare is this? I was truly being cared for and educated in ways I never imagined. This made my journey much easier than it could have been. You all rock! I hope you continue to keep allowing the Lord to use you to save lives and help people to heal. Every nurse, aide, tech, resident, advocate, and volunteer, I wouldn't have made it without your care and diligence. Dr. Rhonda-Henry Tillman (the sound of your clicking heels coming down the halls gave me hope in every visit), you are a beautiful woman inside and out. Dr. Go, Dr. Gardner, Dr. Yuen, Dr. Kent, Dr. Collins, and Dr. Makhoul, I salute you all and the hard work you do every day.

To all of my family members who played key roles in doing any and everything that I needed done and things I didn't realize I had gotten. I actually had a rap song written in my honor complements of my cousin Marcus. That was the sweetest honor ever. I got a gazillion aunts, uncles, and cousins who were very present and very much a blessing to me. I love you all, and you will never really know the gratitude of how much! I had a family of nurses (real ones), cooks, babysitters, chauffeurs, errand runners, preachers, and prayer warriors (real ones), cleaning crew, and comedians! May God bless each and every one of you; and if you think you have never gotten anything else right in your days of living on earth, just know the moment our paths crossed, you hit purpose right on the bull's eye! I would not be the person I am today without each one of you!

XOXO
Sharon

# INTRODUCTION

Do you remember that one fight that you had in school with that one kid? This kid was twice your size, mean, and clearly ready to give you the business. Well, I sure remember this kid oh so well. If you can recall the memory of your thought processes right before the fight, get it in your mind's eye and go back with me. So imagine all the fear, shame, doubt, embarrassment, and plan ole defeat for a moment. Although these emotions were real and strong, there was a slither of tenacity and hope that would not let me run away. I couldn't give in regardless of the feelings that you would lose because you knew you couldn't beat up the person you were about to fight. The only thing you could think of was how small you were and how big they were! I had never had a fight before outside of house fights with my younger brother (who would beat me only if he hit me in the stomach). Speaking of that, even after I was able to regain strength enough to fight for the win, I would come for my brother so fast and take him out! I love my brother dearly, but we literally had fights. Okay, back to the "proverbial Bluto" (please remember Bluto). Okay, so now it is on! You are in the fight, scampering around, tripping, swinging and missing, getting up, and getting hammered! Okay right, so you are probably thinking, why you don't just stop and run away. I wanted to prove to "Bluto" I was not afraid (a fat lie)! But I stayed in the fight, and I even fell down but jumped back to my feet and continued on. I was also thinking, *If I can just get one good landing punch in, things could go in my favor, and I may win this thing.* So I did what any young girl in my time did, I windmilled it

11

out until it was finally over with. I know that technically I was not the winner, but at least the defeat in my mind was gone because I mustered enough strength to change my strategy. This was big news because nobody knew I would even give it a go. As hilarious as it is to tell this story, it is very important to understand the underlying story being told.

Well, this is exactly the experience I had to relive but, of course, in a very much different way. On March 2, 2010, I was told the biopsy came back positive for stage 3 breast cancer with three positive lymph nodes. So here we go in for the fight of my life, a whole journey of pure fight. I, my husband, and our three boys had just been thrown into the ring with this enemy called cancer. Some of the occasional thoughts in my mind were, *Oh, how can I possibly beat this?* I have never heard of this one being something that was a part of my family's medical history. I had not smoked anything since my unruly college years as a sophomore. I was not a health nutritionist or exercise coach; but for the most part, I thought I was pretty healthy. I was a pretty healthy child growing up and was not sickly. Why would this be something I had to deal with? Do I need to have chemotherapy? What does this mean? Will I die? How will my children handle my death? Will my husband marry a good-enough woman to help raise them? What happens if I have to remove my breast? These questions and thoughts plagued my mind with many others day in and day out. Can you imagine?

I was twenty-nine years old, had just bought a home. My oldest child was only eight. We were about to celebrate seven years of marriage, and we were just enjoying life. As you read this story, imagine yourself, your family, friend, your neighbor, your enemy, your coworker, or that lady in the grocery store. Cancer has no limits or requirements on age, race, sex, socioeconomic status, class, religion, or anything else. Neither does it show favor. It is only as vicious as you allow it to be. Don't give up living your best life because you may have faced a season of trials. As the old saying goes, "Put your big girl panties on!"

# WATCH NIGHT SERVICE

IT IS THE END of the year; and I am sitting quietly, enjoying the testimonies of those who spoke so passionately about all the many blessings that the Lord has given them. The overcoming of trials made me feel at peace about my own place in life. I cried silently and thanked God as I thought about how my next year would look. I had always been a person of few words and absolutely hated speaking publicly in large crowds. The first time I remember speaking as an adult in church was when I was in college at my old home church in Dumas, Arkansas, and I had to deliver the welcome for a program. I thought I would pass out. Never mind the fact that the whole church was loving and kind, mostly family, and everybody thought I was sweet girl. Why was I so afraid to talk in front of people? I have no idea. All I know is I sweat profusely. My voice trembled, and I couldn't even read my own writing without missing the words; I think they were moving about on the paper actually. But I finished it; and every since then, I knew I was no good at that. *So no thank you to public speaking,* (so I thought!) God sure does have a grand sense of humor that is unbelievable.

However, as I sat there, I heard a still small voice, "I want you to go into the next year on a fast." And I am thinking to myself, *I am really losing it now, buddy!* In my mind, I'm thinking, *Okay, really, did I just hear that?* I had never really submitted myself enough to do a fast, but I accepted the assignment without reservation. And I was determined to finish it out with the help of the Lord. I sat there all alone and wrote down what I expected God to do for me since I didn't know why I was too fast. He did not give me an explanation. So I just decided to make it out as a request for God to answer some questions for me that I needed to know. I had an actual list of questions for God to answer for me. I didn't ask for money, cars, and shopping sprees. I needed to have His instructions for my life.

Meanwhile, I prayed and meditated daily, and I studied the word. I expected the Lord to mold me into who He wanted me to become. I knew I was an amateur in this journey, but I wanted more of Him. The innocence of a pure relationship is priceless. He surely meets us where we are. Amen! This fast was indeed a process for me; I was very determined to commit to my yes. It was hard, and there were times that I forgot about a particular food item. It would be a close call, and I'd have to hurry to the trash to discard it. I did not want to displease the Lord. I didn't have a team of people to encourage me and a big support circle at this time. My husband was my accountability partner, but he was not into it and thought I would surely slip and fall. However, he would encourage me and pray with me whenever he knew I was getting weak and discouraged. I did a twenty-one-day fast and didn't eat anything but fruits and vegetables. I drank water only and prayed as much as I could. I found strength in quiet times mostly because whenever I moved around, it felt like I was moving in slow motion. I was a praying young lady, learning what it means to have a personal prayer life. The focus was only for me to know the Lord and hear Him clearly. Honestly, I found myself to be very easily moody and uneasy, so I wanted everybody to stop and acknowledge my process and let me be in peace. This is hilarious to me now, but I didn't understand many things. And I was trying. It was hard; I could barely stand loud talking or sudden movements. I was being broken in my flesh and didn't realize it. During this time of consecration, I was at a regular prayer meeting, and that is when I had an open vision.

# THE VISION

On JANUARY 19, 2010, I was at my church, Canaan Christian Center in Pine Bluff, Arkansas, at a regular prayer meeting which is held on a weekly basis. I was sitting down with my eyes closed in prayer; and all of a sudden, I saw myself stretched out in midair and wrapped up in a long white cloth draped over my body. It looked like I was on a long rod being turned over and over again very slowly. Please try as much as possible to see this. Have you ever seen in person or on TV a whole pig being roasted outside over an open fire, almost like a rotisserie chicken turning...? Okay, so this is what I looked like except that I wasn't burnt to a crisp or disheveled at all. As a matter of fact I was very well put together. I was so relaxed and almost looked asleep, and my hair was long and straightened with a wet look. But my whole body moved as one unit like I was suspended in midair, but underneath me was a huge vat of oil in black kettle pot. Inside the pot was hot boiling oil, and it was over a big fire. I was literally being dipped with each turn downward. I was being put into this oil and back out again. It's almost impossible for me to explain what I was seeing. I didn't understand it at all. I was completely in awe of what I saw, it was fascinating to me but puzzling. The next thing I saw was a huge white ram, it was standing in the back of the church peering right at me and I remember the horns were shiny golden, but the most profound thing was how white it was and it wasn't moving only staring at me and then it vanished. The only person I told at the time was my husband. He kind of looked like I was cray cray, and I couldn't blame him. But I knew it had to be a significant thing I saw. He was astonished at how vividly and passionately I was explaining what I saw, but he was clearly not sure of it. I must have sure come off my rocker. Eventually, the emotions of it all wore off, and time went on. This memory will be with me until I am no more; I had never experienced anything like this prior to that night at prayer. Surprisingly, I didn't think of it much, and it was way in the back of my mind. It was a few months later, and I had a very strong memory of the vision as if it was happening again, and I know precisely because it was my 30th birthday. That's when the Lord explained it all to me.

Note to self: Always ask the Lord to increase your understanding and your trust in Him with the vision.

# THE DECISION

## RECAP TO SEPT 2009

Eᴀʀʟʏ ᴏɴᴇ ᴍᴏʀɴɪɴɢ, I began my normal duties for a busy day, but today was going to be different. I knew it in my heart. I was about to make a decision that I never really wanted to make; but at the time, I was thinking immaturely and a bit impulsive. My heart was always for my husband, and I to have at least one girl and one boy. Believe it or not, actually the original plan was to go for six (three boys and three girls). Life began to happen very fast, and our numbers went from six to four and then three and then back to four and three again (you will soon see why). By the time, our second son was born. We knew we wanted to have a girl without a doubt. Every mother likes to proclaim that she knows the sex of with her child before she has the ultrasound. So it was a great shock to me when I found out the little girl was not happening yet again. Certainly the third child would be a little princess. It was an emotional time for me knowing after finding out that even our third child would not be a girl but another boy, so we decided to possibly try again. But the timing had to be right for us (whatever that means).

> *Prayer: Lord, help us to be thankful that we are able to give life. I don't want to be selfish. I accept your will. Do what you want to, Lord. I need to be free in my mind from worrying over the wrong things. Will I ever have a girl, or should I stop trying now?*

Anyway, the Lord knew what we needed even when we did not! At the time, my third child was three years old. And I really wanted to have one more shot at it. It seemed that every other month, I was having symptoms, and we were on a constant emotional roller coaster only to find out we were not pregnant. We were trying to conceive but not really trying. I know that makes no sense to most, but somebody knows what that means. It was always mixed feelings because we wanted to plan everything all out. Not knowing if we had succeeded unexpectedly would be too much to handle because we knew when the perfect times would be to conceive (these were our true thoughts). Therefore, every other month, literally we were buying pregnancy tests; I know I was paranoid because sometimes we were using the POAP method! (stay with me, you will know what this is soon enough). I know we are not the only married couple that struggles with this situation! Stop it right now and own your truth. Okay, honestly think about it. We are young, vibrant, active, and very frisky couple. That is what I will say on that point. God is good! There was a slight conflict for me because as a married woman, I felt bad by wanting to have contraception. What is the alternative here? I knew eventually we would find a good stopping point, but how do you make that decision seriously? I had reached the recommended childbirths due to my previous surgeries; otherwise, there would have been a strong chance of complications above normal. The choice to make those decisions without someone else giving the demand was not what we wanted to hear, so we wanted to try again. But after so many failed attempts, we knew it was right to move on. As parents, that needed to be our decision. We told God if it is meant to be, we trust the outcome. However, we didn't really mean it. Our actions were a mess. As I share with you the narrative of how the conflict gets resolved, you will see in the following dialogue:

## The Conversation

September 2009

Me: Hey, baby, do you remember after Anais (our third son) was born what you told me?

Alex: No, what did I say?

Me; You never remember.

Alex: What did it have to do with?

Me: Okay, so you told me that instead of me having a tubal, you would gladly volunteer to have a vasectomy. Remember how I told you that you will never have that done, right?

Alex: Oh okay, baby, you are right. I'm sorry. I'm going to make an appointment soon.

Me: Boy, please it's two years later. We have had too many pregnancy scares, and I have decided I'm going to the health clinic get some birth control pills.

Alex: Birth control? Nooo, I don't think that's a good idea.

Me: Well, I don't either, but you know what, I wanted a little girl. God didn't think we needed one, so I'm good with my three boys.

Alex: But you said you didn't want to do that.

Me: I know, but you lied to me. And I have made up my mind. I have already made the appointment.

(Quietly walks out, thinking to myself, *This is crazy. Why should a married woman take birth control? I shouldn't be on the pill, the shot, or anything.* But I'm not changing my mind.

Alex: Okay, well, I guess you know what you are doing. Whatever you decide, I'm okay with that.

Me: Yeah, I bet! Well, this is better than getting my tubes tied (tubal ligation).

## OFFICE VISIT

Doctor: Hello, Mrs. Rejistre, so what brings you in today?

Me: Okay, Doctor. I'm married, and I have three children and a dog. My husband and I are satisfied with our family, so we just need extra comfort knowing that we are taking precautions from another pregnancy.

She then proceeds to ask all the medical history and ask what form of protection we had been using so far. And I paused for a minute and told her POAP. I knew she didn't know what I meant, and she asked, "What is that?"

I was so excited to tell her. "It means pull out and pray!" She let out the biggest laugh ever, and we had so much fun in that moment. But it was the truth. We finished up with the exam. She asked me about what contraception did I want, and I asked for a Mircette (because I had previously used it and had no weird side effects). But that particular one was no longer on the market, instead offered me Ortho Tri-Cyclen Lo.

Me: Okay, that's fine. I will take that one.

Doctor. Okay, great, I'll be right back with them.

Okay, here you are. Is there anything else I can help you with? If you have any questions or concerns, give us a call.

I left the visit with my bag of goodies feeling happy. I did not begin taking them until the Sunday after my next cycle began, which was only a week away.

Prayer: Lord, forgive me for this, but I don't know what else to do. I would have preferred this to be done in a different way. Help me to get through this. Hear my heart's cry, O Lord.

# LEOPARD SKIN

IT WAS ABOUT MID-NOVEMBER, only a couple of months after taking the pill. I woke up to do my daily routine, and I noticed the first real change. What in the world is this on my body? I lifted my top so my husband could see, and he asked me what it was. I said, "I don't know. I just noticed it. It was not there yesterday." I looked like a leopard on my torso, several small black spots as if I was allergic to something. Standing in front of the mirror puzzled, I had no idea. It didn't itch, or I didn't have fevers or sore throat. I called the doctor's office of the health department and explained what happened, and the nurse asked if I had any other symptoms and told me to take some Benadryl and use Dove soap unscented. Wow, really? It seemed weird and uncaring, but I thought maybe my body is going through changes. I am getting older.

After a couple of days passed, all of a sudden, while in the shower, I felt my left breast on the outside near my arm pit, and it was a prominent hard lump. And that's when it dawned on me, *Oh my goodness, what if the birth control pills are making this happen?* On a Saturday morning the following week, I woke up, and now I'm sore to the touch. I asked my husband to feel it and immediately pain. He told me to give him all the pills, and we were going to the doctor. Well, by this time, I no longer wanted to visit the old doctor, but I went anyway to ask her if the pills could be the cause. She said the rash looked as if it were related to a change with soaps or laundry detergent, not related to the pain in breast. I knew better than that, and I was not about to accept this. So I called my mom and asked her could she make an appointment with Dr. A (in my hometown), who was my doctor for all of my childhood. I was uninsured with no primary care physician. If at any time I was not well, I would simply go to the local health clinic or what we would call urgent care centers. Dr. A was a trusted family doctor, and we all loved him dearly. However, if I had known what was about to take place, I would have made better choices. I had a state job at the time, and we all had the options to make changes to our health insurance policy if needed. I walked my happy self in the room with those agents like a silly woman and cancelled my health plan. I thought about that as I made this next appointment and you will see how.

# FIRST ALERT

THE NURSE CALLED ME back, and I was waiting on some answers. I showed her my concerns with the lump and the spots after answers. I was expecting to do the normal routine, BP, temperature, weight, urinalysis, and etc. However the doctor came on in, and he asked me what was going on. He examined the rash, and then he did a breast exam. He said that he needs to do a needle biopsy. Clueless to the fact, I had no idea what that was or why he wanted to do it, and I never asked. I just knew it would involve a needle. I am not the average person who freaks out about needles, but I also was no big fan. Whenever I had to be poked for any reason, I always looked away. I hate to see how long or how big they are. I agreed to do it; and he left the room, came back in, and explained that if he could draw fluid out, we wouldn't worry much. But if it's no fluid, it indicates a tumor. Again, ignorance had me thinking it was just a small thing that was in the way and needed to be moved. I encourage you to always ask questions always get a clear understanding if you are not certain about things going on with your health or your loved ones. If you need clarity or want to confirm things, ask specific and direct questions. He proceeds to examine and, to my surprise, no fluid. He looked at me and said, "We need to get you scheduled for surgery. We must take it out and look at it"—what?—"I'll have the nurse to come back in and talk to you."

2nd Nurse: Okay, Sharon, the nurse wants to get you scheduled for a surgery. Can we get a copy of your insurance info?

Me: (Trying to understand with a puzzled look) I'm not insured. I am paying out of pocket today for this visit.

FYI: There is no excuse for any person to be employed at a decent job that offers insurance and not take advantage of the benefits. We were recently due to update our enrollment or make any changes to the policies we had if there needed to be changes. I decided to change my policy, opted out of coverage; and ironically enough, I actually had a cancer policy. You know what's even more ironic? I said to a few family members and friends, "I do not need that. I can save those extra dollars for my pay check. It is too much." This was absolutely the true place of where I was. I later understood that I had been living with an impoverished mind-set and caused me to think in a low place, and therefore my expectations were sort of nonexistent. A great word for anybody out there who needs to hear this: your life is priceless. There is no dollar value worth having over the security of a proper health plan. You never know what you will need. If you don't have a plan, now is the time to get one please. It was bad enough that I had to pay out of pocket for whatever I needed done, creating debt that I absolutely should not have created. But again, you cannot put a price on your health. It ended up working in my favor because we simply did not have enough income to afford the screenings, exams, and care. God had it all worked out even in my ignorance.

Then this really nice nurse looked at me and asked if I had ever had a mammogram or a breast ultrasound before. Can you imagine me wondering, *Now why would I need that?* I explained nicely that I had not, and she gave me some great information about the grant program through Susan G. Komen funding allowed for women who needed their services. At the time, I was thinking, *Oh, that's nice that they have programs like that available.* She then informed me that the same program was available in the current city I reside in (Pine Bluff) as well through the local hospital. She gave me the name and number of the contact person to start the process. I called, and she assured me that one of the top surgeons in the state was the recommended way to go. So I agreed to meet with the Dr. Z, but it would be a couple of weeks before I could be seen.

# THE STATE'S BEST

AS I SAT THERE waiting on the specialist to come in for the first visit, again I must say it never dawned on me why I was there or what were the possibilities. I never asked. In walks this stern-looking man in his white coat and ready to get down to business. I felt like this was a good decision I have made to see this doctor he is going to figure out the problem and help me. He did a thorough medical history and exam, and he asked me about how the area of my breast with the lump was feeling. At the time, it was not hurting but that it was there and just hard lump. The conclusion of this visit was that we would watch it and make sure to see if it just goes away or see what happens. Anybody who has ever been diagnosed with breast cancer knows that this is an ultimate no-no! If I had known then what I know now, I would have not continued this medical relationship. However, most of the time when a doctor is a specialist in one area does not make them good to determine certain decisions for your health when there is much more going on. It does not mean they are bad doctors in my opinion. I believe they are just not informed enough to realize we need to act fast. It is better to be overactive than to be nonchalant. I recommend any health-care professionals out there if you are reading this, never tell a patient to just watch it. We need clarity and answers, not a time frame to watch things get worse and could even mean our very life coming to a rapid end. Be honest with your patient if you are not as informed and then do a proper referral. It could mean you saved a life by doing so. Remember early detection saves lives!

I still didn't expect anything serious to be wrong, so I agreed with this doctor who was one of "the best" in the state. He told me to change back in my clothes and that the nurse would be back in to get me scheduled. By this time, I'm not sure what to think. I was settled with "maybe I am experiencing what fibroid cysts are." Off to home again with no real answers. At that point, I was no longer hurting, and the rash was finally leaving. I have had no other reactions, so I thought I was in the clear.

> Prayer: Oh, Lord, keeper of my soul, will you please guard and keep my spirit throughout the night seasons of rest? You know my cry. Lord, I refuse to give my family up to the enemy. I trust you, Lord, to see us through!

# LATE NIGHT DATE NIGHT

WE WERE AT A church member's house for a youth Christmas party, and we were having a nice date night after we dropped off the kids for the sleepover. We were overdue for some alone time and trying to get back in the groove of just having fun. When the night was over, I remember feeling sick to my stomach again. Maybe I'm finally pregnant (here we go again). It was a sharp-shooting pain. This feels really weird. I had a sudden urge to go to ladies' room, and I sat there. Nothing happened, but I noticed there was blood. That scared me, and I freaked out pretty bad. Wow, we are having fun, enjoying each other's company, no children to look after; and then we discussed that one time, I was late with the pill. A little glimmer of hope stirred my mind. My husband immediately thought it too. We needed a pregnancy test. I was getting excited again only to find out that night, it was negative. But something was wrong; I felt bad and couldn't explain, so I automatically assumed that I had a miscarriage. The test could have been faulty. We went to the ER; and the final report was that if I was pregnant, the hormone was not high enough to detect. But it doesn't appear that you were pregnant. Neither of us knew the specifics of it all, but this was another sign of seeing things going wrong in my body and not knowing what to do.

*Prayer: Lord, I hope I am not being punished for taking this pill. Should I stop now? We decided we were okay with our three boys. I will trust you, Lord.*

The doctors said it wasn't likely a pregnancy. I am getting older. My body is changing, and maybe I'm just adjusting to the pill. We were at least able to dress up and go for dinner and a movie, no kiddos, and a clean house. There is hope for us to date we just needed to get our friends to keep our boys.

# THE WAIT IS OVER

THE DOCTOR HAD INFORMED me at the last visit to "wait, let's watch it," and we come back in thirty days unless something happens. As I stated before, I trusted the doctor's plan and recommendation. Remember I had no reason to suspect anything. Well, at about the twenty-third day, I started feeling the lump more prominent than before, and it had gotten bigger than before. It began hurting to the point of going without wearing certain clothing and my bra. I wanted to call and go to the doctor early, but I talked myself out of it. I wanted to follow his plan of waiting; and by the way, I was only a week out before the whole thirty days were over. But my husband strongly urged me to call sooner once I finally explained to him how I was feeling. Word of wisdom: Please tell your family what is going on with yourself it is unfair to withhold information. If you experience anything going on in your body that is not the norm, please get it looked at right away.

On the day I went back for the follow-up, my husband was right there with me. Every process was superfast. I was back in the next day for the surgical biopsy. By this time, all the proper paperwork was complete for the Arkansas Breast Care program. (Thank you, Dr. Josetta Wilkins. You are a real boss lady.) I had no reason to wait long periods for anything, so I went back in for the results shortly after the the-same-day procedure. I can remember my husband asking me that day, "Babe, do you want me to go with you to your appointment today?" In my mind, there was no reason for him to come.

I replied, "I bet it's nothing. I'll be okay. It's just those cysts that women get all the time. You go on to work. No need in missing too many days for nothing." We kissed each other and parted ways. I walked in the front door. The nurse called me back before I could turn around to look for a seat.

"Sharon, you can come on back." I entered the room excited to get back to my day and started my daily chores at home, and this wait seemed like an eternity. I was checking emails, texting my friend, looking at Facebook; and almost thirty minutes into waiting, Dr. Z walked in.

Again, he was serious faced, holding his clip board looking down at my files and saying, "Your test results did come back positive for stage 3 breast cancer with 3 positive lymph nodes, blah, blah, blah, and now I'll have the nurse come in and get you set up for your treatments right away." By now, my eyebrows were in the middle of my forehead. I was confused at what I just heard and tried to figure it all out, and the nurse, a kind lady, walked in. She said nothing. Instead, she reached out to me while I'm sitting here on the medical table, and she hugged me. We said nothing to each other.

These couple of minutes seemed to last so long, and she embraced me. Then I'm not sure what happened but it felt like someone hit me in the stomach, and my body was suddenly very limp. I said it. "I have cancer." The tears rolled down my cheek, and that's when she released me.

She said, "Blah blah blah aggressive blah blah blah chemo blah blah blah blah choices and decisions..." I'm not sure what all was said for a span of about thirty seconds, and then she asked, "Are you going to be okay?"

I replied, "Yes." And she said she can go ahead and set me up to meet with Dr. Y and get started with treatments right away. I said, "Yes, that's fine."

"Okay, you can go ahead and grab your things. Just call us if you have any questions, but we will call you later today with your appointment day and time."

When I walked out the doctor's office, I know now I was in shock, but I called my husband right outside the office. All I could say was that they said I have breast cancer, and I need to start treating right away because it is aggressive. And again, some weird sounds were coming, like Charlie Brown was in my spirit, "Mwa mwa, blah blah blah no second opinion mwa mwa mwa, this can't be true."

"Call your parents and your aunts." This is not an exaggeration. We literally had a conversation that I can barely remember other than he wanted me to have a second opinion, and with all the energy and force I could, "IT'S MY BODY, MY CHOICE. AND IF CANCER IS IN MY BODY, I WANT IT OUT NOW! NO SECOND OPINION! THIS IS AN EXPERT!" Although I did not like his bedside manners or attitude, I was willing to stick with him and get the ball rolling. Well, I love my husband dearly, and I do trust him. So I did at least call my aunts (Renay and Marcia); and after all the mwa mwa mwa, I was not going to have a second opinion. I didn't realize at the time how much this meant to my husband, but he wanted me to be sure if this is what I wanted to do. He asked me to repeat everything that the doctor said; and I think what affected me more was his attitude, his demeanor, and manners more than his words because he didn't seem to care that he just told me that the life I had known prior to that visit was over. And I would have to hit the brakes and find a new way of living.

I don't remember what happened next; really, it all had gotten fuzzy. I remember calling my parents like I always do every day. When I repeated what the doctor said, it was as if I had never heard it before. Listening to myself say the results was deafening. I felt like my ears went out or something. Silence and then they both began talking positive. I am their firstborn, and we were always being goofy and talking on the phone all the time. They had no idea the news was coming to them at all. The normal laughs and pitch of their voice on the other end of the phone didn't sound the same. I didn't want to tell them, but I knew I had to. I didn't make a big deal about all the signs and symptoms before. If I had known, I would have shared everything and would never be passive. I never connected the dots that this could be possible. I had a mammogram, ultrasound, and biopsy. It was true. I had breast cancer. We all had just been slammed with a ton of bricks on the edge of a very small cliff!

# THE SECOND
# OPINION

**I**T MADE MORE SENSE to do the second opinion to me even before anyone said anything. I was not feeling good about how I was handled in that very important appointment. I would have valued some empathy and concern from my health-care provider. I urge all providers to be mindful that you do this kind of work every day, and you may possibly become mundane. But it is necessary to show compassion. I also knew I was not going to waste much time to start my treatments, but I absolutely wanted to make sure I considered my husband. I just didn't know that I would agree with him on this one.

I was at work, and I got an unexpected phone call from Dr. Joanna Edwards. She was one of my old college professors, and we developed a close bond throughout the years that transcended the class. She had a conversation with my husband earlier that day at his office, and he informed her of the tragic news just received. She is such a kind and soft-spoken lady. She called me while I was at work and asked would I mind going to lunch with her. She wanted me to meet her sister who was a breast cancer survivor for over twenty years. I honestly did not want to go, but my respect for her and the genuine concern for me was the encouragement I needed to say yes. At the time, I had an hour lunch, so I knew it would be good enough time to get back to work soon. I stood outside, speaking to myself, "Lord, I do not want to do this. I just want this to all be over with. What is going on in my life?" She drives up so fast on the parking lot, and it gave me a slight chuckle before getting in. We greeted each other with a hug and few words. The ride in the car was mostly quiet, but we got to a beautiful brick home not too far from the University of Arkansas at Pine Bluff. I slowly walked to the door; and this smooth-skin elderly woman, full of grace, greeted me with kind eyes and a warm smile. As I walked in, I felt the presence of the Lord; and I began weeping again, sitting there on her couch. Dr. Edwards began to explain what was going on, and Dr. Wilkins began to explain to me her personal story, as well as her professional story. The most important piece for me at the time was the way she placed her gentle but firm hold on my hand and looked me in the eye and told me that I would live. Life was not over. I had decisions to make, and it was no time to be overly emotional. But I had to think with purpose. She had her own triumphant victory to share and agreed that a second opinion was necessary before I agreed to go further. I explained that I didn't want to prolong the wait to move forward. Immediately I was able to witness the favor she had with the best surgeon that I know, Dr. Rhonda Henry-Tillman, and was able to get an appointment the next day. I was again overwhelmed with emotion but this time of joy. It was a blessing for a stranger to encourage me and offer to extend her support and the referral for a second opinion.

The day of the second opinion, I was nervous and hopeful, wishing there was no cancer. The results were congruent with the first results, and she took time to explain to me exactly what was going on according to the results and another exam she did in office that day. She comforted me and educated me about the disease and what it was showing in all the results. She was very polite and wanted me to be at ease with my next decisions. By the time the visit was over, I knew I was not only there for an opinion, but I had just met my new doctor. She was hired, and the other one was fired! She was very personable and even reassured me that she would do all she could, gave me her best medical advice, as well as personal advice, because I asked her to. She did not sugarcoat anything, but it was her care and bedside manners that encouraged me. She came in the room, smiling big each time, regardless of what was happening, and it became contagious. She gave me so much insight and wisdom about how to properly care for myself and make ready for the upcoming changes. My husband was right there, and she accepted his opinion and made him comfortable as well. It was not long after that, and I began my first treatment. She introduced me to most of the medical team before we had our first official appointment. I prayed from day one until my care was complete, when I knew I would be in her care. Any and everybody who helped me physically were on my prayer list! I needed heavenly wisdom from the Lord to get through this journey. It was weird things that I found comfort in while visiting my doctor. The sound of her shoes were loud and strong. She wore actual heels and clogs to work, and it made me feel like I was not losing my femininity. She made we want to care again about how I look. I was thinking, *What does it matter; I will soon be a disfigured person.* I had been told that I would have to remove the breast tissue, and I knew the possibilities with losing my hair. I just didn't want to care anymore. Although to have the second opinion was a good idea, it only confirmed the reality that my life would never be the same; and that part, I did not like. The best part of it all, she listened to me and allowed me to have a say in what was happening.

# MOM HAS CANCER

IN A MILLION YEARS, never did I ever think I would have to explain such a complex and challenging thing to tell my kids. I was sure that I would tell them before I lost hair, before taking treatments, before they would witness me staying in bed, not picking them up, unable to clean and cook. I wanted them to be ahead of the surprises. I didn't know how to explain this to them, but the Lord did! My husband wanted to tell them a lot sooner than I thought of, but I knew it had to be done without too many emotions. My children are born in the "SpongeBob," "Teen Titans," "Kim Possible," "Fairly OddParents," and a "Jake Long" kind of generation. They loved all of those shows and then some. The cutest thing ever was when I introduced them to a few of my generation's cartoons, and they loved them. One in particular was Popeye. I was praying about how to tell them, and then it came to me. Bluto was a mean bully who wanted to beat up on Popeye. Popeye was the little guy who didn't stand a chance with Bluto because he was bigger and stronger than him. Until one day, Popeye eats his spinach like we all do because when we eat our vegetables, we get stronger, and our bodies can grow like it is supposed to. Well, I told them I was like Popeye; and until I get my spinach, I would be beat up by Bluto. I explained that Bluto was this thing called cancer. It was mean and bad, but I had the strength to fight back. But I need to take my treatments just like the spinach. I told them it would make me look a little different, and I would get a little weak but only for a little while. I had to have a lot of spinach and rest. This seemed to work very well with them, and I was excited about the Lord's creativity. But I was not prepared for the next question. My oldest son, in all his wisdom, looked at me with those big brown eyes and chubby cheeks and said, "So does this mean that you are going to die?"

In this moment that felt like a lifetime, I held my face and smiled, "No, son, this does not mean that at all. I am going to be fine."

"Oh okay, that's good. Well, if you want to talk about it, we can talk about it later." We hugged; and I went to my room, turned up my TV, and buried my face in the pillow. I cried and screamed. I told the Lord that day, "I cannot leave my kids. They need me, and I need them. Please don't let me go." Little did I know, I was speaking life over my situation in spite of how it was looking to me. I would always do whatever I had to do for my boys; and in that moment, I needed to be alive! I am so thankful for how this worked out in our favor. That was a hard thing for me to figure out how to tell them.

# MY CO-SURVIVORS
# ARE THE BEST

It is an honor to have a network of people supporting you, encouraging you, and caring for you. Whatever capacity someone gives their love, please receive it and do not take it for granted. Now is a good time to establish where boundaries are needed in relationships, whether it is spouse/partner, casual, work, spiritual friends/family. Take out a pen and pad and quickly write who would be on your first list to notify in case of crisis or emergency. These are probably considered your support system, if you didn't realize before. No negativity or Debbie Downers allowed. I do apologize in advance to you; but even if, it is your relatives who can sometimes be negative. They may not have meant to be that way, but you will know even now as you read this if "that one" comes to your mind, wink. Yeah, do not add this person to your support system. They could be of help in other ways but not in your inner circle. Keep things in perspective as to who you need to ask to be your support if you need it. Most importantly, those that do not have a strong prayer life/faith walk would not be of any good as to pray firmly for healing in what may appear to be a life-threatening concern. Perhaps you are not sick or never have been sick, but you need to have good people in your corner.

Message to caretakers: maybe you are the caretaker. I want to sincerely take this time to say thank you from the heart! Your loved ones need you too, that they do not want to be vulnerable, dependent, and helpless. It takes a lot of humility and strength to allow the process to unfold in a healthy manner. We need you to get your own support circle as well. Sometimes the support system needs to focus more on the co-survivors than the actual patient because, at least, we (patient/survivor) are being treated physically; we have a lot of attention. I recognized it, and that was hard watching my husband and boys suffer the pain and agony of not being able to help me get better, in ways that they wanted. Be encouraged and get the help you need. We do not need to know everything at the time. But get some trusted believer to support you in your process. In the same way, you need us; we need you to be healthy and well.

I would not be the person I am today if it had not been for this gruesome process. In a strangely weird way, I am a better person than I was before. Cancer is something that should never be welcomed or praised. It comes to take you out; but if you ever find yourself dealing with it in any way, you have to make it work for you and your family. It is okay that what works for one person may not work for another. There is no exact path to figure it all out. Trial and error, things work, and then they don't. All of my family and friends, I love you! My mom and dad took the time to help care for me, hand and foot, in any capacity. My words will never be able to express the appreciation for what you have done for me and my family. I am blessed to be your daughter. I could say so much, but I save it for our multiple phone calls (that we have daily)! Once I received those three dreaded words, I never realized the details of what would be needed. I don't think anybody knows at first all of the details that go into having people around to do for you, especially family.

People, listen up. Your family is not obligated to do anything, and there is a willing decision and sacrifices that goes into this. I literally didn't have to ask for anything—well, maybe just that one time. Brace yourself. I had to call my cousin, Mary; and boy, did she deliver! Listen, constipation was a real problem, and it had me emptying my whole purse to see the manifestation show up! Whew weee! I remember that day like no other. Pain medicines on a continuous basis had me unable to go to the bathroom, and I am so grateful for my little cousin, who was in college at the time, right down the street from where my house was. (Kisses and hugs I send to you, girl). I love you, Mary!

Okay, now back to what I was saying. My entire family seemed to have sat down and mapped out a complete plan to pitch in on this process. I had coordinated rides to doctor appointments when my husband had to finally go back to work and couldn't make every single appointment, but he was very present with everything going on. The doctors and nurses had no problem speaking to him about what each visit was like and any other information that we needed to know. I could not rely on memory alone, so I would write things down. But if he needed clarity, they provided the details. Everybody was there, supporting me in one way or another, supporting my well-being. There were people (in addition to family) who cooked large amounts of food continually (Ma Joe and Big Sis Cheryl). It is a pretty vulnerable place to be in when you cannot cook for your own family, but it was soon okay because I was being pampered and taken care of and so were my husband and children. The aroma and smell of food being cooked at my home were horrible. Almost everything made me want to puke if I could smell it. It had gotten better over time, but initially we learned it was better to cook it away and bring it in. I had tried so many pills to deal with chronic nausea until we found the magic combination (about three different meds). All of this can be hard on a patient's senses; I literally had to have a milk jug gallon that I had cut off the top of it, so I used it adequately every day all day to keep with me around the house.

God provided enough help for us that everyone seemed to work in cycles except my mom. She worked tirelessly all day until my husband came home from work at night. Now all of this sounds wonderful, right? Well, yes and no. I'll explain. Well, when you are accustomed to being the one to do so much and care for everybody, it is not easy not being able to do the same. I felt guilty about my family having to do this for me. I wanted to be well. I would tell myself every day, "I will show them how much I am thankful one day." There was a new level of humility at this time and no room for pride.

This place of vulnerability made me emotional most of days. It was admirable and a blessing. We had family and friends to cook, clean, help me do my hair and bath. I was unable to drive anywhere for a while; so once my husband went back to work, we did not have to worry with anyone picking up our boys from school or even after-school babysitting sessions. We had really great help, prayer warriors, cleaning the house, and running errand. We were being blessed financially, as well as many other things.

Another example of a co-survivor coming to save the day was the day I cut the straggly strings of my hair. Christopher (my cousin) and his wife (Belle) came to my rescue. I was so embarrassed at how my hair had thinned to baldness in some places. I woke up one day and decided I had to comb my hair for the last time. It was devastating. With every stroke of the comb, I would see so much hair, and I cried every day. I had enough of it and wanted to take what last bit of control I could muster and make it work for me. I called and asked if he would come and cut it all off even; and without hesitation, he came. He smiled so big, showing all thirty-two and looked at me and repeatedly told me how beautiful I was. His sweet wife said, "Sharon, girl, you are so beautiful. I know you don't believe it, but it's gone be okay and get you some big earrings. You got the perfect head for the cut."

I was like, "Oh, okay!" I was not feeling it at all. The irony was that I couldn't wait to go wig shopping again; but this time, it would be because I felt like I needed them to feel better about myself. Back story to this irony:

> *A month before I was diagnosed, our church had a Valentine's ball. I had found a cute dress and gotten my nails done. But I waited too late to get my hair done, and no one could get me in before the event. I almost cancelled, but my husband was excited and had gotten a nice "churchy suite" (laughing so hard right now). My pastor would've said he was in his "Sunday go-to meeting." The thought came on my mind to go get a wig. I waited too late to schedule an appointment at the beauty salon and my hair was a mess, now anybody who truly knows*

*me would have thought I was crazy because I was very verbal about not liking young woman who willingly wore wigs on a regular basis. My thoughts were that it makes no sense to wear wigs when you have hair and under a certain age. Well, I was in a very different space. It felt weird, but I was open to it. I started trying on wigs, and it was fun. I found one that I really like, and it seemed pretty close to what I would actually wear. Bingo! I found the perfect wig, and we left in a hurry to the ball. This was the beginning of me actually liking the wigs prior to be diagnosed. I just love God's sense of humor! It worked for me, and I am glad it happened that way.*

I sat there and quietly. Tears rolled down my face, and all I could think of was how silly I am to be this sad about hair. The reality is when you are already dealing with certain insecurities with self-image, it was like second nature to be overly consumed with hair. I was hopeful all the way, until I lost my hair, that I would be one of the women who would not have to deal with hair loss. It was possible; but in my case, it was just a matter of time. I met a beautiful lady (who will remain nameless, I'll call her Lady T) during my third or fourth chemo treatment, and she encouraged me. She said nothing I wanted to hear, no pity, and no beating around the bush. We had the exact same diagnosis, the same doctors, and the same treatment plan. She was at the end of her treatments, and I was just getting started. She informed that around the second-week mark, I would start to see a lot of hair shedding. I remained confident that I would not be that person; but just as she said, there were patches of hair gone. One morning, I woke up to see long strands of hair on my pillowcase. We talked several times after that, and she even gave me a small prayer cloth. I felt as if an angel had visited at my bedside that day.

We do not get to pick and choose what message the Lord will send; but right when we need it, the answer is always there. I didn't like the message, but I was thankful and was able to relax when the physical changes happened. We were immensely blessed, and it was overwhelming at how everybody put aside their needs and allowed the Lord to use them to help me and my family. I cannot say enough thanks and praises. There really is not a separation of positions after people go through this with you; you realize your family is much bigger than blood alone. There were key people who may not have come over to my home or a doctor visit, but they were at the feet of Jesus and thought enough of me to fast and pray for me. I say to the ones who fought for me when I couldn't fight and stood with me in spirit, you are the MVP. I had an amazing support system.

I also have to make mention of one of the best organizations around, Living Beyond Breast Cancer. I love you and all you stand for. You gave me the hope I needed to push me into advocacy, to ignite in me the vision of Pink Orchid and to reach back for every other women faced with breast cancer. The cancer conferences literally helped save my life. I absolutely consider LBBC as my support system. There were so many people who I developed friendships with, people from all over, and some of us are still in contact today. If you are in need of additional resources and information, group support, and network opportunities, please look them up, not only for patients/survivors but also for health professionals, as well as family members, governmental officials and legislators, and other community advocates. There is a plethora of information for research, funding, advocacy, awareness, education, training, and good old fun times, as well as other information for those affected by cancer. I want people to realize the importance of having an effective team of support, big or small, is vital to recovery and healing. There will be complications, and some adjustments will need to be made. But key people can provide a safe community well balanced enough to get the patient/survivor on a good path.

# EMPTY THE BAGS

My husband and I were being very well taken care of with a family full of nurses (literally four licensed nurses). I had no need of a home health aide. I had a double mastectomy with reconstruction and an axillary lymph node dissection. That just means that I had both of my natural breasts removed and implants put in. (All of this was done on the same day during a nineteen-hour procedure). I also had a few lymph nodes taken out of my arm because they tested positive and needed to be gone. How in the world am I going to be okay? As I was headed home after surgery, I wondered what this all meant for me. There were a few things to take note of to ensure I would care for myself properly, have a positive outcome, and have a speedy recovery. I know now that I wasn't the best at caring for myself, but I did learn. I followed instructions; but most of all, I prayed like never before! I had to take my pain meds, take care of bandage sites, rest, and empty bags. I know for certain I had many instructions, but this is what stands out most.

The day came when the cycles of visits for cleaning, bandaging, baths, and getting in and out of bed was coming to an end. My family had to, at some point, go on with their lives and allow us to do more and not handicap us. We certainly did not like this part and was very accustomed to their presence and help (okay, we were being spoiled). My drains were draining more slowly because I was better and had no signs of infection. One evening, after realizing I should have someone to empty them, I didn't want to bother anyone to come over, so I waited on my husband to come in after work and kindly asked, "Now, baby, it is your time today. Can you please help me to drain the fluid?"

And without hesitation, "Nah, sweetheart. I'm sorry I can't do it. That's too much on me." Surprisingly he stuck to his word and did not do it; I was for sure he would do it. Can you believe it? My husband did not want to empty the bags?

Now, I was not aware at the time how devastated he was to see me this way. So I said, "Oh, I'll call the nurse," with attitude. He did apologize, but I realized later it wasn't easy, and he was a little grossed out at all the tubes, fluid, and the appearance of my surgical sites. He thought that he would mess up; so I had to read my notes, call the nurse, and take my time. Before long, I didn't need any help draining and cleaning the areas several times a day. I was in pain most days from surgery, and it took a while to do everything. But with time, it got easier and a little faster. My favorite thing about having those drainage bags was a cute custom waist apron. It was very convenient, and I liked that more than carrying a bag around. I finally found a nice enough bag I could tote around if I was away from home; but at home, I preferred my apron. The inscription was "ABCs and DDs" written on the front of it, and it had three big pockets large enough to hold them without complications.

I hated the idea of walking around with tubes hanging from me. It was uncomfortable, and I just hated it all. Although I was in the house unless I was going to doctor appointments, I still thought it was a bit much. I felt like snatching it all out and sleeping like I would normally sleep. I had to be extremely careful because a few nights I freaked out when I woke up when I felt some of the fluid on my gown. At one point, the awesome pain pills I had allowed me to sleep so good that I snapped one of them out by mistake, and I had to call the nurse. Thankfully, she told me I could call an aunt (Marcia, Renay, Chris, and Rosemary, thank you so much) who came over to reinsert it because it was pretty easy to do. I thought for sure to myself, *My boob would definitely leak out and deflate, and I would need new surgery.* I had no idea how silly this was; but at the time, this was all real in my mind. I had gotten pretty good at cleaning the sites and draining my bags, thanks to my husband, who simply didn't have the stomach for it. This drainage wasn't so bad after all. Thankfully my surgery incisions were so clean/neat, and my aunts and the nurses at my follow-up appointments would always complement how good they looked (this was so weird to me), and how well I was doing was shocking to them. Those words were somehow helpful and encouraging in the middle of getting better. We do not realize the true power of words until after the fact. Every little bit helps and can really transform the outcome of a situation.

It seemed as if I was smack dab in the middle of eternity and that my body was taking extremely long to heal. Ironically, my medical team all agreed that I was healing at a rapid rate, and my initial scars and incisions were actually nice enough to get a smile out of me. When I took my very first shower alone, I had no drainage almost. and it was time to go back to the doctor to get them removed. Yaaayyy! I was so excited; I knew I wouldn't feel like a science project anymore!

# CLOSET ENCOUNTER

DURING THE PROCESS OF being a cancer patient, I adjusted to the highs and lows of each day, the side effects of meds and the doubt and fear very present through most of my treatments. Yes, it is true. I am a believer in Christ that struggle at the time with thoughts that plagued my mind. It wasn't the ideal thing, but it was pretty normal day-to-day, not knowing pain awaits and what questions my family would have if I would feel strength coming back in my body or if I could stomach today's meal. There was a night when I woke up to agonizing pain; it was approximately 2:00 a.m. (I know this exactly because I took notes in my journal.) Pain radiated my body all over. And I couldn't scuffle fast enough to the closet. I tried to move as quietly as possible. I didn't want to wake my sleeping husband. My husband worked so hard at making sure our home was as comfortable as could be. Bills were being paid, and the kids wouldn't be worried about anything else. That first night that I was awakened I couldn't help but to pause for a minute to look at him and lightly stroke his head, whispering silent prayers, "Thank you, Lord, for him. He is not perfect, but he is just right for me. Please keep him safe and strengthen him daily."

I walked to the master bath. I got the pain pills and throw them back. Shooting sharp pain makes me cringe even now. Literally tears began to flow. I almost crawled to my bedroom closet (it was big enough for me to lie down in) for prayer. I sat in there. It was pure darkness, silently weeping and praying for relief and lamenting. I cried out, and it seemed as if my voice escaped me and traveled off. As clear as ever, I saw a bright light enter my closed closet door and a hush paralyzed my cry. The pain was gone, and joy filled my heart. I lay down on my hand-woven blanket, praying and now crying tears of joy because I knew heaven showed up for me. I had never experienced this before, but I will never forget that moment. It seemed as if time stood still, but all of this occurred within a span of an hour. Quietly, I made it back to bed and kissed my husband and listened to his horrible snoring until sleep came again.

Song by Walter Hawkins: Thank you, Lord, for all you've done for me! This song is what I was singing within myself many days after the visitation. Now many would say how could she sing a song or be thankful in a situation like that? Well, time was passing. My thoughts became clearer, and faith grew stronger. It is no lie. Having cancer sucks really bad. The surgery is agonizing. All the meds are annoying. The pain gets unbearable, and the whole situation is disrespectful! But I was breathing. I had family. I had a vision, and I wasn't ready to tap out. So to encourage anyone with any obstacle, I say to you, "Find the beam of hope while you're in the midst of your process and make it work. Don't give up!"

It's supposed to be because it is. (Targie Crumpton)

Prayer: Lord, bless all of these people who are taking part in helping us. Bless all of my doctors and nurses. They are so kind and patient and never make me feel like a nuisance. (I asked so many questions.) I'm sure I was on edge about different meds, tests, and symptoms, and side effects.

# HAPPY BIRTHDAY TO ME

I WAS ABOUT TWO MONTHS into my treatment, and I remember this so clearly because it was my thirtieth birthday. I had another strong memory of "the vision" (pause and read it again). The Lord explained it all to me that day while I was literally hooked to the IV. "I have already prepared you for the process of what you are going through. It is the anointing of the oil that keeps you. You will come out of this better than when you went in. Do not be afraid you will live." And that was all I heard. That's it. That's all.

Do you know how long it took for me to really understand and feel the power of that word? There were many days and nights filled with agonizing pain, tormenting thoughts, feelings of doubt, and almost every side effect you could imagine when going through chemotherapy, radiation, and surgery. I was very much saved before this process started. I remained saved during this process, and I am still saved now. None of those things negate the fact that I was a human being faced with a real process that I simply didn't welcome or even want to complete. Lord, how is this making me better? What is the point in all of this? How long will it last? Yes, even after knowing and believing I would be okay. I want to encourage every person reading this. No matter what your issue or your trial may be, it is okay that you may struggle with your soul-ish battles. You will have questions. However, be assured in your faith and trust that you are simply in a transitional phase of life of temporary situation. Do not allow any-

49

one to force you to deny your humanity. This is my story and realize the truth is we all have times where we struggle with the reality of our now versus the truth of what is! Lord knows I was lost in the mix of it all, and I thought I was broken. I thought, *Perhaps my faith is not good enough. Maybe all the bad things I had ever done came back to punish me.* I never thought that God was punishing me, although I have friends who said that is exactly how they felt. Every patient and/or survivor has the absolute right to feel how they feel; but as a believer of Christ, I realize the conflict this may cause and even how others may seem. But with the proper support system (this includes a diverse group of people), with prayer, and a wholesome care plan, it will most likely be improvements of health.

What was the significance of the oil? Why did I look like I was being cooked over an open fire but I seemed to embrace it? Nothing made sense to me. It was the power of God that kept me through it all. Eventually after the fog cleared, I had to make a decision with clearer vision to accept what God allowed. It doesn't mean it was breeze, but it was definitely worth every day. I was able to keep going. The oil is definitely costly! In all that I went through in this cancer journey, I was encouraged by the price our Savior paid through His death, burial, and resurrection! Hallelujah, you can make it! Glory to God!

# THE BEST GIFT

IN THE BEGINNING, I wasn't too happy because on my thirtieth birthday. I was taking a four-hour treatment. The Lord had just explained to me what I saw, and a million questions went through my mind. The explanation made me at least feel comforted in knowing all will be well. The unknown place is a place that is uneasy. I believed that I would be okay, and healing was my portion. It started out pretty ridiculous. All I wanted was to be healthy and not be in the place I was in. Being angry and sad only made things worse. I should have focused more on what really mattered in the moment, but I did not. I felt justified to be mad. Hindsight! I am still a work in progress, but I learned so much about myself. I was at least open for the Lord to deal with my heart and show me because I asked.

It was in my cancer journey I found out I was a selfish person. Does that sound mean or not? I love the Lord; He made all things plain when I began to ask. Although I didn't understand everything, He did tell me. I wasted many days on focusing on the negative instead of being thankful for the time I had. I know, being human, we make mistakes and are not always aware of the good things to be grateful for. I was alive and able to have a birthday; but because it was chemo day, it felt ruined. If I could have had one true wish during that time, it would have been to at least have strength in my body to get away with my husband like we would normally do and travel. Of course, looking back, I would have changed much of that day except my sweet surprise birthday dinner. Little did I know, my husband had made plans for me in spite of everything and arranged a date on chemo day. He surprised me with a late-night dinner date at Cantina Laredo. He knows how much I appreciate a good Mexican dish. I had finally gotten a healthy appetite, and I was ready to devour food every second of the day. The medicines and remedies I was taking at the time helped tremendously to support an appetite. I wanted to eat so bad. I didn't care if it was healthy or not. If I could hold it down or even have the desire to eat, I went for it. So we are at dinner, and he began to shower me with gifts and making a big deal because my day had consisted of being at the hospital until nightfall. He had already made plans and didn't tell me anything, which is rare. He can barely keep a secret because he gets excited and tells it all. It really ended being a perfect night, especially since I was able to eat a meal! I cried like a baby and was so thankful he was with me the entire time and never complained.

I didn't understand much about what it meant to make faith confessions. I equated it to faking it until you make it. In the beginning stages of this way of living, I couldn't grasp the concept. It felt very disconnected and disingenuous to confess things that were not yet so. I was simply stating what the bible stated concerning healing. I learned that getting into agreement and reaching for it (healing power) when it just was not available or manifesting. Regardless of my feelings at the time, I was building my inner man and learning how to agree with the Holy Spirit about my healing. I felt crazy. I really believed it was somehow possible and hoped that maybe I can benefit from it; I just kept on confessing in faith. I was tired many days and wondered why am I still here and why did my friends have to die. It was as if guilt began to set in. I knew I was unworthy, and I know I had done nothing special to still be alive. On this journey, if you are blessed like I was, you meet so many amazing people, who fight and win. Some have more challenges than others, but their stories are all inspiring. It is like a brand-new family you become part of. Of course, you don't want to be in this family, but you are. You figure out a way to make it work and encourage each other. The tragedy of loss of friends and family hurts really badly, and it takes time to grieve the loss. I found that in this process, I would deal with occasional thoughts of bitterness and fear. This is important because I didn't feel like it was fair that I had to have so many friends I had made were soon gone. and then the tormenting images of death and everything surrounding my life felt like it was spiraling out of control. Honestly, I would even say to myself, *Even my friends would not have to deal with the whole fight of cancer any more.* I had to slap myself back to reality and shout "thank you, Jesus, for keeping me here. I haven't done enough living for you yet."

My pastors at that time was Apostle Craig and Sheryl Banks. They were such a godsend to me and my family. A few days after my birthday had passed, I had received a text message that read: "Hello, WOG, I got something for you. Make sure you see me after church. Love ya much!" Now I was thinking, *Oh, okay, maybe I got some fruit or water. They are so sweet.*

I replied, "Okay," and didn't think too much of it. It was not a big deal; she would send text messages from time to time to encourage me or just to check up on me. I really didn't realize she remembered my birthday. It is a challenge to remember the details of when I got the gifts from her, but one of the best cards I ever received reads: I apologize for the late birthday, but this makes it extra special because this is the only one gift you get today (and yes $ was included). It was all about the message. I loved it, and I thought to myself, *Now that's cute. I am going to get late gifts from now on for everybody so I can say this same thing to people!* It was genius. That made my day because it's true, and it felt good to be thought of at a time of such chaos and pain. The gift that was the icing on the cake was *God's Creative Power* gift collection, a small leather book by Charles Capps. Oh my, this was a real game changer for me. I am a person who enjoys reading anyway; but when I begin to thumb through the book, I could literally smell the anointing oil. Either she prayed over it and blessed it, or my senses were extremely wide open in the spirit. Perhaps both of these scenarios were true, but either way I was super geeked. I loved the title. It was a cute book, and I had never heard of it before. I will plug it forever. Please go add this book to your personal library. It is a must have if you are looking to boost your faith or need healing, or maybe you are look-ing for a gift for a loved one. Get this book!

I didn't feel much when I first started reading it, but it was a good read. I was not going to stop until I finished it. I would think to myself, *This is a good book. It is very powerful. It has a lot of Scriptures, and it makes so much sense.* But that was about it. I knew I needed to keep reading it. I was talking with Pastor about it, and she suggested I just keep reading it. And I did. I finished the book pretty fast, but I kept reading it. I believe it was about the fifth time; and it was near the beginning of the book as I begin to read, something hap-pened. I cannot really explain it, but I will try. We had taken a trip to Maryland to visit family, but my aunt had also asked if we could take my cousin (Kaneidra) along for a campus tour in Hampton, Virginia. She would soon be attending Hampton University. I did not know why this bright young lady would want to come all this way from family to this college, but we loved her and supported her every decision. I was excited for her. After we got her there and found out where she was supposed to be, I sat in my car and waited on her return. I pulled out my book, and I can't remember exactly the words that I read in that moment. But I literally felt like my insides quiv-ered as if I had been hit in the stomach, and my bones almost felt like they were being fed. Now, I am aware this may sound ridiculous to some and silly to others, but I must stay true to the experience I had. I felt an overwhelming joy came over me and guess what? Yes, I cried. The Holy Spirit resonated within me, and I began to receive every word of what was being said. I was now onto something! I began to read this book like my life depended on it. There were no new words. Nothing exciting happened, but a flood of peace came over me. I had never felt this way before. I loved it, and I wanted more. So I would still read it from time to time just because I knew it made a difference in me. I have no idea how many times I've read it, but it was definitely in good use.

Several years after this experience, I met another survivor through a friend, who became very dear to me. I felt led to pass this book on to her. I did not want to, but the Lord wanted her to have it. She has transitioned home, but we had a special connection. And she expressed to me before her passing how much she needed this book. I was thankful she made a peaceful transition and was blessed by "God's creative power." That was enough for me.

# MY AUNT AND MCDONALD'S

Most of all my family went to Detroit, MI, in the summer of 2010 for a family reunion. I was super emotional and upset that I could not attend; but of course, I did not admit it to family. I would not want them to miss out on their fun times to sit back home with me and watch me be sick. That would have been a little selfish, so I agreed that I would be okay. I honestly thought I would be okay with the exception of being emotional. I was home with my three children, no adult company, not really enjoying my time. My husband had gone back to work, so he wasn't home. The children were busy playing games, watching TV, and horseplaying as usual. The problem for me was that our family has always been super close, and we always did family functions and outings together. But here I was at home during the summer months, beautiful day out, but I was stuck indoors. Some days, my husband worked on the weekends, and this was one of those days. I finally decided enough is enough, so I got out of bed (probably too fast) and called for the boys to get cleaned up. We were going out for the day. My treat to them was McDonalds; and of course, they were excited. I grabbed my wig and my purse; and just as I opened the door, there was my aunt. She was reaching for the knob when I swung open the door. I was startled of course. She stood there, smiling with her two grandchildren at the time. "Woooe, you scared me. Where did you come from?"

She said, "We are coming to see you. Where you going?"

I then told her I thought she was in Detroit with the rest of the family. "You caught me. I'm busted, auntie! Listen, I'm sorry I didn't want to be in the house."

"Where are you going? It's okay. We will go together." Now she didn't even pay attention to the fact that I probably did not need to get out of house so early after a chemotherapy treatment, but I was just excited to see the sunny sky that day.

"Okay good. We are going to McDonalds."

"Okay, well, you know I couldn't go with the family either. I just got out of the hospital and didn't want to take any chances of anything getting worse."

"Oh yeah, that's right. I forgot about that."

On the drive over, we had a pleasant conversation of which I do not remember much of. The moment I stepped outdoors, I was consumed by the beauty of everything and was feeling immediately better mentally. What I was thinking about all that day was how we take for granted the small things: the nature, birds flying, little children playing in the distance, the hot beaming sun on our skin, the way we are able to see how vibrant colors are, how fresh-cut grass smells, and again family. It was pretty hot outside that day, but I did not mind it at all. I had probably, at this point, six or seven treatments, and it just seemed like an eternity. The days and times were running together, and I would often times have to ask what day it was if I didn't have my phone close by. Well, this day was about to get even more exciting, and it all started with me wanting to sneak out of my house to get some time away with my boys. It was important that they saw me having fun and hanging out like we would normally do (prior to cancer).

Special note: My aunt is a Licensed Practical nurse and has been for almost thirty years. She was literally surprising me, her sick niece, that day for some time of fellowship. I know now that she was a true godsend that day at McDonalds. I want you to know if you are a cancer patient/survivor, please do not leave home alone too soon during treatments, if you can avoid it. That could possibly be very dangerous.

McDonald worker: Yes, may I take your order please, ma'am?

Me: (Looking down at my phone) Yes, I'm sorry.

McDonald worker: Oh, hey, Sharon, how are you?

Me: (Putting on a good face as if I know the person's name but I didn't. I did recognize his face because we had psychology courses in college together). Hello, how are you? I'm doing okay and you? Okay, good, so let me have blah blah blah.

McDonald worker: Okay you look so good. It's nice to see you. Is it for here or to go?

Now in my head, I'm thinking, *Dude, seriously I should just snatch this wig off so you can be quiet with all that.* But I played it cool and smiled. He was not flirting at all; he was always a nice guy and was being his normal self.

Me: Thank you. (By now, I am noticing I need a seat.) It's going to be for here.

My aunt then proceeds to the counter and makes her order; and everything was going fine, not a very long wait at all. So out our food comes, and we head for our table. Then as soon as I sat down, wooosh! I felt extremely dizzy and weak. I started sweating profusely, and I rested my head for a minute on the table. My aunt asked, "Are you okay, Sharon?"

And I replied quickly, "Yes, ma'am. I am fine. I'm just a little hot." As soon as I said that, I jumped up as fast as I could and ran for the bathroom. One shoe came flying off and the wig. I kept running to the toilet; and before I made it there good, I was vomiting all over the place. I puked my guts out and then nothing! When I started to come back around, I was in the ambulance. My aunt was talking in the background. I could smell the vomit on my wig; and as it hit the side of my face, I could feel that it was wet. I still had my eyes closed. Can you imagine how embarrassed I was? Nope, I bet you cannot. Well, I came to myself, and my husband was there holding my hand. All these thoughts were going through my head, *Where did he come from? Who called him? Why did I get sick? Did they put the blood pres-*

*sure cuff on the right arm? Oh my goodness, these people saw my wig fly off. Where are my kids, and where is my shoe (still didn't have it)?* All of that and some. I was simply too weak to start talking so much.

> Prayer: Lord, please teach me to be patient with myself, to love myself, and to relax. I thank you for my family and the angel you sent for me today.

This was not the easy day it was supposed to be. I did not intend on ruining a perfect day out with my boys. Now imagine if my aunt had not showed up in the nick of time. How would that day had gone if she was not there? The chemotherapy treatments are draining; and if you are not careful even on your "good days," they will leave you passed out on the bathroom floor—with no wig, one shoe, and in a pile of vomit—after a seizure. My aunt later informed me that she rushed to my rescue in the bathroom, and I was having a seizure. Word to the wise, when it's hot outside and you are a current cancer patient, just stay home inside and relax. I am for certain that I may have not had that episode in the comforts of my home because I would have been in bed resting as I would normally do. But the fun doesn't end there. I was checked in to the local hospital. I do remember the doctors and nurses were so kind. They got me hooked up to the monitors, IVs, and I had blood drawn. One of the ER nurses walked in, and I remember her explaining I need potassium very badly; my numbers were too low, so I had to get the drip started. I was eager to get back home and ready to get whatever I needed. Boy oh boy, I was not prepared for that IV dose of potassium.

Nurse: Okay, sweetie, you might feel a little uncomfortable, but we have to give this to you.
Me: Okay

All the while, my husband remained at my side; he was a sweetheart then and still is now. He laughed and talked to me about why I was out of the house and fussed a little but was relieved that I was doing well. We laughed about it a bit, but then I felt this strong sting-ing burning feeling in my arm.

Me: Baby, please tell them to come get this out of my arm. Something
    is wrong. (I was already pushing the button.)
Husband: (Runs out to get the nurse and explains what was happening)
Nurse 2: Oh, ma'am, your drip was going a little too fast. I'm so sorry.
Me: Please make it stop. How much longer do I have?
Nurse: Oh, you have a lot left. We can't let you go just yet.

By this time, the sensation had already subsided, and I was already feeling better.

Hubby: We have got to get you some bananas and potassium supple-
    ments. (I hated eating plain bananas; I only liked them in my
    mom's banana pudding.)
Me: Okay, I'll eat whatever I have to. I don't ever want to do this
    again. Is this normal, ma'am?
Nurse: Yes it is. Potassium doesn't feel good going in. But you have to
    have it or, your body will try to shut down on you. (She walks
    out and encourages me to relax.)

I remember my husband caressing my bald head, and I drifted off to sleep. My husband was trying to whisper on the phone, speak-ing to my mom. I couldn't make it all out, but I did hear him ask her if she wanted to speak to me. By now, both eyes were open, and I was peering at him. He smiled and handed me the phone.

Me: Yes, Ma'am?
Mom: What are you doing, Sharon?
Me: Getting some medicine.
Mom: Girl, you gone make me hurt you. You scared me. We are way
    out here in Detroit. Take care of yourself. How are you feeling
    now?

Me: I know, Ma, I just wanted to get out of the house with the boys. I miss y'all, and it was so pretty outside. I feel better now. The freaking potassium was hurting, but they came in and fixed it.

Mom: You know better than to do that. Well, you better make sure not to have them hurting you. I know Reggie is going to make sure. Okay. I love you, baby. Let me speak back to him

Me: Okay, luh you too, Ma.

A couple hours afterward and the visit was over, and we were able to go back home. Moral of this story is just stay at home and rest!

# SEVENTH YEAR ANNIVERSARY

DISCLAIMER: THE INFORMATION IN this chapter is considered for those mature enough to handle marital affairs. If you consider yourself to be a super saint, this section may offend you. I am not responsible for any offense and weird emotion you may feel due to proceeding or any other thing you do not like. I apologize in advance, but this is real life.

I am a country girl who enjoys long car rides, traveling all over the place. I get just as excited about the actual drive as I do about the destination at times. Oddly enough, my husband decided this year, we would celebrate in Tulsa, Oklahoma. I was not too thrilled about the destination; but it was close, not too far away. Besides, I was leaving my home and the state. My doctor was not excited about me taking the trip and recommended we stay close to home. Even though, at first, I was not thrilled, suddenly my excitement was at its normal peak. The color of my skin was coming back, and I had just bought a new colorful maxi dress. My face was dolled up (this generation calls it a beat), and I was ready. This was one of the few times I actually felt pretty after cancer. We stopped at our hotel room as soon as we got there, and it seemed as if we were rushing to our room. Of course, my husband wanted to immediately bless the room (wink, wink). We absolutely did just that. In the heat of the moment, I'm trying to stay cute and all dolled up, but then he snatches the wig off and threw it across the room. We both laughed so loud, and I couldn't believe he did that. This was especially funny because, during my cancer journey, he was nice and gentle with me. But those days came to an end that day. He had been gentle long enough and had no intentions on playing nice!

We got ourselves ready to go out on the town, freshly showered, clothes ironed, and I had drawn my eyebrows back on and reapplied a little makeup. The only thing I needed was my wig, and we were ready to leave. I started looking for the wig, and it was nowhere to be found. I looked everywhere. I looked on the floor, on the table, under the table, behind the TV, under the curtains, and in my bags. He joined in with me looking everywhere I looked and still nothing. It had to be somewhere; we didn't turn around to see where the wig landed at the time. I sat down and started to wonder, *Maybe it's behind the mirror.* But when I got there, I saw in my peripheral a black shadowy thing. I turned and looked to my left, and it was right there inside of the lamp. It landed perfectly on the light bulb. The problem was it had been there too long and melted a hole right through it. "Oh no!" Immediately I began to cry. I didn't know how a wig can burn that bad but because it was a pretty cheap one and it was literally on the light bulb as if it was on one of those mannequins' head. I was never a person who was good at judging wigs and didn't know much about them because normally I would not wear a wig. I thought they were for elderly woman. However, I had grown pretty attached to my wig. It was probably only about $20; but out of all the wigs I had, this one was my favorite. I did not bring a second one on this trip.

Finally, my husband tried to console me and said, "Let's just go buy a new one. We can get whatever you want to replace that one." He told me we can find the nearest store on my phone, and I did. "You will be okay." I did not like the idea of going out bald; I had never gone out without a wig.

I was working up to being okay and said, "Let's go." I got the GPS and pulled up the store, and we were on our way. The hair store, to our surprise, did not carry any wigs for women of color. What! This whole scenario was getting worse and worse. We drove around and didn't find another one.

We stopped and even asked a few locals, and no one knew where I could go. Finally, he said, "Look at me. You do not need it. You are beautiful just the way you are. Please, we need to celebrate and enjoy our trip!" So I wiped my eyes again and forgot all about hair and wigs. I even took a picture of myself smiling in front of Oral Roberts University, in front of the big praying hands. I was still sad at that point; but when I looked at the picture, I was smiling so big I tried to not feel the shame or the embarrassment. It was a really good picture. It meant something special to me to be there because I had heard the story of my maternal grandmother who had visited this very place before she died. She had the privilege of meeting Oral Roberts, and he prayed for her. She was a cancer patient and transitioned this life at an early age. This was the day that I decided I was truly not defined by those wigs, my bald head, or any other thing that would prevent me from being free.

> Prayer: Lord, thank you for my husband. He never changed on me. Help me to see me how you see me, Lord. I need to be okay with who I am. This is a difficult process. How long is this going to be this way? I am grateful that my husband sees me as a whole person. Glory!

# HERE WE GO AGAIN

ONE YEAR TO THE date of being diagnosed, March 2, 2011. I went back in for a checkup because of pain. We were thinking the surgery was causing changes, but it was, in fact, a reoccurrence. Yes, that is correct; on the same day, I was diagnosed a year later. My favorite doctor examines me and immediately sets me up for a new round of chemo and another surgery. I was absolutely shocked at the news, but I was no longer the same—the fear was gone, doubt was gone, that negative self-talk was gone. As we sat there in the exam room, my husband's breath was heavy, and his face was sad, but I grabbed his hand and said, "No, we are going to beat this."

The words that my doctor spoke echoed in my room. "I don't know why this cancer is back. We gave you the best treatment plan we had. We can give you another round of chemo, but it's not as strong as what you had before, and we have given you the max amount of radiation. We can take that cancer out through surgery, but it is really close to your rib head. We will have to see if we need to remove one to make sure it's all out. It's no guarantee it's going to work, but we will try."

Can you believe this? This new sounds much worse than before. But I told my husband, "It's okay. This time, we know God is the one that gets all the glory, not the treatments, the doctors, or anything else. He will do it!"

The time I had spent in the Word of God and in my secret place with Him had perfected that steadfast hope. I had developed the mind to speak life. My perception had totally changed, and I knew all was well. I received a call after a few days, and my aunt Marcia and sister friend Cheryl were visiting, and the nurse said that the cancer had not penetrated to my ribs, and I would not need to remove any. My nurse informed that chemo was still needed as well as surgery. I agreed without hesitation and praised God all at the same time. I have many thoughts about this process, but I will save that for later. It is a joy to know when God has done a great work in me, and I remained full of peace. Even though I had a second attack with cancer, I only celebrate my first cancer-free date. God does not make any mistakes, and when He said I'm healed, I believed it. He didn't change His mind on me. So I held on to the truth instead of facts. All with help of the Lord, I made it out again. The devil tried it, but it didn't work.

# FROM THE OUTSIDE IN

As A SURVIVOR, IT is a very real notion to understand how important it is for family and friends to receive support and an outlet to express their concerns and emotions. Proper perspective is needed so much after dealing with the mental turmoil and the side effects of the treatment. This is one of the most important chapters in this book because the strength and support of loved ones helped maintained sanity and hope. So this chapter is a viewpoint from my spouse, my parents, my oldest child, and my best friend. Healing had to come full circle for my new normal to take place. The idea came from God while cleaning my floors, and he told me exactly who was to contribute to this chapter. It was good to be instructed on this matter. This chapter would have undoubtedly been the longest because so many dear to me could easily share how their life or our relationship shifted. The meaning of this chapter is for you to have a small viewpoint of how it looked from the outside in. There is much fuzziness (chemo) even now about the details of emotions and thoughts shared of this process.

Dear co-survivor,

It's okay to be vulnerable and communicate the honest place of what was in your heart and mind. This particular section will hopefully strengthen many others who are co-survivors and caretakers. It will also give some sort of therapeutic release to bring healing to families and even the survivor. I am very much alive. I am not a robot or super human, and I am not serving a life sentence. I was anointed for this process. God knew all about this! This is life now, and we are going to make it. We don't have to know all the answers, and none of us like it at all. But it is what it is. So let's do life and make it happen!

## THE HUSBAND

When my wife, Sharon, was first diagnosed with stage 3 breast cancer, I immediately equated it with death. I equated it to death because at the age of eight years old, I witnessed the death of my stepmother. The death of my stepmother was very disturbing to me because of the things I heard from my siblings concerning gruesome surgeries she had to go through in order to fight back for her life. Even though these surgical procedures failed, it still left me with horrible thoughts and to hear my father cry. I can still see the engraved picture in my head as I write. Even though I did not spend a lot of time with my stepmother, the experience that I witnessed my siblings and my father go through shaped and molded and stabilized the feelings and thoughts of my wife's final fate at that time, thinking back on how unstable my father's household became, with my siblings having different women in and out of the house after my stepmother's death. All these thoughts started racing through my mind from time to time like, *Who would help me with my kids from a female companion standpoint?* I mean I would go to church or be invited to speak, somewhere and my flesh would say, *What woman in here would possibly be a good fit for you when your wife die?* I was truly in a state of "this is it." Where would I move to with my kids to try and cope with the death of my wife? And finally, how can I shake my mind to believe God's Word that he would never leave me nor forsake me? I know all of this sounds strange; however, nine months prior, I had lost my mother after talking to her one day before the last four weeks I would ever talk to her again.

The devil had me so confused, thinking my life was never going to get stabilized from this death spirit. I truly was in a state of panic because my business had started failing due to some prior complications that resulted in me losing over 65 percent of business revenue and the rock behind my business death eight months post to my wife's diagnosis. I was once told that deaths come in threes, so my faith was really shaken after all of this. In the beginning, following my wife's diagnosis, we had so much support from family, friends, and survivors; but after about three to four weeks, it was the immediate family: me, Sharon, Alexander, Aaron, and Anais. We were the starting five for team Rejistre, and we all worked as a team to try and support one another. It's hard when you're an alternative physician; and death is knocking at your spouse's door after taking your mother, office manager, and trying to take your wife. But he that is in you is greater than he that is in the world (John 4:4). Therefore, no weapon formed against shall prosper through Christ Jesus. We are more than conquerors.

Once I started building up my inner man and reassuring my wife the same, we started to be very closed off with just allowing any person around our home and who we were communicating with, especially after my son came home (Alex) and informed us that one of his childhood friends informed him that his mother was going to die because she had cancer. There were so many things I remembered that affected me, but the day of her first surgery was hard. I was unsure of what to expect following such a major transformation as this. A bilateral mastectomy, I have to say initially it turned out great! I mean Dr. X did his thing, and my wife rocked her new C cups! Although I heard former cancer patients say, "Blame it on chemo," I surely thought it was a term used in a joking matter; however, joking was not allowed much in our home at this time. I had to deal with a reality of my wife not feeling like herself again and only having mirror images of her past self in sporadic episodes. Now if these words were just for small talk, self-realization or to make me feel I should not want to be with her was something I had figured out in less than five seconds, and my response would be "of course not, my dear, you are beautiful." Now granted, of course, my wife didn't look like the little hot dumpling she did in college at UAPB, but there was no way on God's green earth I was going to say that. I remember it like yesterday. My pastor told me to tithe on what I'm believing God to do in my life following my wife's sixth chemotherapy treatment. I just wanted my wife to be healthy and live! The phrase that still echoed out to me is "putting God to the test" (Malachi 3:10–12)! Let's just say all these years later, God is still holding it down!

## OLDEST CHILD

As a young boy, finding out that my mom had cancer, I did not understand the reason for her sickness. The only thing that caught my attention was her going bald. Seeing my mom go through something like that only gave me one thought and question in my mind, and I asked her "Are you going to die?" But as I asked my mom with a curious tone of voice, she told me without a worry on her face and made it all better, but sooner things had begun to change. My mom had to take a lot of medication, take a lot of trips to the doctor; and we had to lose our family dog, Sammie, because my mom couldn't be around her while taking treatments. A lot tears were shed, and it was a lot of confusion roaming in Rejistre household; but through all that, God told my mom "I got you."

## DAD

My daughter first told me she had went to the doctor for a lump on her breast. And the doctor told her there was a chance of her having breast cancer. I would not claim that in the name of Jesus. As she went back and forth to the doctor for tests, the doctor confirmed that she did have it. That was a punch in my stomach. But I know I had to be strong for her when she began her treatment. I did my best to encourage her that everything will be all right. When the doctor told her that a certain time that her treatment would be over, that was when they came up with something else. I had to watch my baby grow tired of all them different treatment. I being the father, the head, the protector, it was nothing I could do for my little girl. So I went to my secret closet and prayed for strength for her and me because it was wearing me down to see her go through that, but I couldn't let her see that. You can't imagine how that felt. Many nights of tears I cried. But thanks be to God my prayers were answered. My baby is cancer free and has been for some years now.

## MOTHER

This is a brief summary of what I was dealing with when my daughter was diagnosed. These things happened a few months after she began treatment. It was as if someone had turned on a water faucet one day; and everything came out all at once but in stages, if that makes sense. Just sitting here, thinking about my oldest child Sharon M. Hudson Rejistre at the age of twenty-nine years young, fighting breast cancer. I cannot turn it off. My life turned upside down when I got the news. It felt like my heart was in my throat, and that feeling stayed there. "Lord!" I cried out. "This chain has to be broken in the name of Jesus!" I called my pastor Reverend JL Morton; but I talked with his wife, Sister Iris Morton (a sweet godly woman). I told her the news and asked them to keep my daughter in their prayers.

She said, "You know we will." And then she asked me how I was feeling about it.

Crying, I answered, "I'm fine." All I can do is pray about it. I couldn't really tell her how I was feeling. I would've fallen apart if I had started to talk about my feelings. *Lord Jesus*, I thought to myself. Sister Morton let me know that they were here for me even if I needed to talk or anything. I knew every word she spoke was the truth.

Now at the time of treatment, it was hard watching my child get over a treatment and witnessing what it had done two or three days after. She was sick, weak and could barely eat anything for days. Just as she starts to feel better and gaining a little strength to eat something, laughing, and pressing her way, it was time for another treatment. It starts all over again, all the pain and the thoughts, the conversations I was having inside. (When I am so weak, but God!) I felt like I had to be strong. I couldn't let her see anything less in me as her mom.

One night, I was home cleaning, singing, and praying. I was all done, and I sat down at my computer. I was feeling fine (at least that's what I thought). I was all alone, can't really explain what I started feeling, but I said, "Lord, what is this?" The tears welled up in my eyes, and I started to rock myself from side to side in that chair. Tears were just falling; I picked up the phone to call my husband but no answer. Now the tears were really falling, and I called my sisters, Chris, Marcia, Shell, and Flo, but no one answered the phone. My face was wet with tears streaming down. (The pipe done burst.) Now I was a mess and in full sob mode, and in a loud voice, I cried out: "Jesus! Jesus!" Rocking and crying, I saw something coming so fast a few feet in my hallway from where I was sitting, a white robe and his feet. I felt him put his arms around me and instantly so much peace. Those tears became tears of joy, no longer sad or heavy. The burdens were lifted off of me. Thank you, Jesus. His presence left, and then the phone rang. The tears were still flowing, but they were tears of joy. I answered the phone, "Hello."

On the other end of the phone, she said, "Hey, my favorite cousin."

I laughed a little, "Hey, Irene." By my voice, she knew something was wrong with me. She just started to encourage me. I just listened to her; but when she was done, I told her it was the Lord that had her to call me. She said she didn't want anything else. She just called. I said I know; but before we got off the phone, we both were laughing. A great release is what I needed. That night, my sleep was so peaceful. I knew everything was going to be all right with my child.

He (the enemy) lost that battle, and he tried again. I stood in the gap for my child at the altar one night in revival, and the Holy Spirit set upon me. Thank you, Jesus! I know it would be well!

After, she was finally cleared, and the doctors said it was all good. She had to go back in for another surgery because they said the cancer came back. I said, "No, it did not!" The cancer was there, but I said that's what they missed. It was already there. They just didn't get it all out the first time. They were saying they may have to remove a rib out. Well, they were talking devil talk. So I called my pastor again, talked with Sister Morton, told her what they said, but I wouldn't say all of it. I asked them to keep praying. I was playing it all over again, over and over, in my head the things the doctors were saying. I was praying and encouraging my daughter and her husband. I had to be strong. Sometimes I couldn't even respond to people at church. I couldn't answer my sisters or brothers when they asked about Sharon because I was trying to hold it together, but they understood. God never left me. I just knew that he was talking to me still through Pastor Morton. This was weeks after she's back home even when she was done with all of this. One of my pastor's text messages: "Things are not always the way it looks, and whose report will you believe?" I'll never forget them for this, and it was months later. I said to God, "Lord, I hear you."

I could have taken off running. Pastor J.L. Morton and Sister Iris Morton, I love y'all with all my heart and thank you, church family! And Dr. Alexander Rejistre, my heart went out to you too. I saw you; I saw your pain, your heaviness, and your tears. But you did exactly what a godly husband should for his wife, kids, and your work and your home. I couldn't talk with you at the time about it. You needed encouraging too. I want you to know love you, son.

## Best friend

I'm writing this with tears in my eyes. When Sharon told me she had cancer, I didn't know what to say or how to feel about it. I had multiple things going through my head, me thinking selfishly and negatively, *What will I do with her not being here? Who will I tell all my secrets to? Who will understand me like she does? Who will finish my thoughts like no other person in my life could do?* My heart felt as if some of the veins had become discounted. Then I, still thinking negatively, I'm like, *I'm gone have to really step up and get a bigger place to stay, so I can help Reggie with the kids. So I can help pick up from school and sleepovers, to give him some peace and quiet for a change because I know that's what she will want.* I can remember her telling me several things about what was going on with her. She once asked me to speak at her funeral. I told her I didn't want to talk about that. I knew I wouldn't be able to talk. I'm like, *She is not only my best friend for over a decade. She is like the big sister I never had.* My heart was crying. As time went on, I'm like, *Why I am I being so selfish and negative? I got to be in good spirit. If she is not negative, why am I?* I can remember her losing all her hair. She still had a smile on her face. I was like, *Oh my god, what a strong, virtuous woman.* I could only imagine how she was feeling. If she was feeling some type of way about how life is and how her life was, I never saw it. I always heard her speak life into her situation in addition to praying. I do feel that she is very blessed woman with all the support and love that she received from her family and friends. By God's grace and mercy, Sharon is alive and well. I thank God for saving my "lil" yet big sister. Love ya, mwah!

# WILL I WORK AGAIN

CANCER IS NOT A death sentence in the way that people once thought of long ago. Cancer, in some cases, gives a person an opportunity to recreate life. I had the worst time ever after the diagnosis, treatment, surgeries, and radiations. I tried to regain strength and confidence to go back on my job (state of Arkansas) at the time, and it was far too soon.

I have heard of many success stories of women working while in treatment or even after treatment, so I was ready and willing. However, the embarrassment of falling asleep on the job, dizzy spells, and (the icing on the cake) falling out in the bathroom in a pool of vomit while soaking in sweat, I figured I needed to go home and rethink my recovery. Of course, my doctor agreed I did not need to work any time soon, and possibly I would have to put work off all together. This was one of the most depressing times ever. I had just met one of my great friends and prayer buddy (Shenetta). The job was not hard, really cool, and able to help people, talking to people every day (one of my strong suits).

Suddenly I ended up getting into a cave of complacency and boredom. Wondering if I would ever find my niche at a career, I tried a few things, but nothing happened. I enjoyed the job, but it wasn't fulfilling an inward desire. I always knew I wanted to be my own boss; but whenever it came to helping others, it was a good fit for me to work a job until the right time came. The creative genius in me began to come forth like never before almost all day long, ideas, projects, activities, events, and whatever you could think. I was mentally going 100 mph while sitting in the bed most days. I shared a thought with my BFF/sister since 1998 TLC to try and compare what I was feeling, and I told her, "If you can close your eyes and imagine the most biggest volcanic mountain in the world and it is at boiling point of eruption but at the very top of the opening is a gigantic steel lid with a deadbolt lock on it, strong enough to keep the lava and eruption inside. If you can see this, imagine this is what I feel like. I am the volcano ready to explode and do the natural process of releasing what's inside. But because of issues, limitations, and whatever this lid is on my life, I am unable to move forward." This was as clear a picture I could paint.

Her response was like, "Wow, oh my god, sis, that's deep."

And I said, "No, that's real." As a word of caution to anyone reading that may have relatives or close friends, be patient with your survivor. Everything has been turned topsy-turvy, and finding the ground was not always easy. This is where I am inserting an extra shout out to my husband; he supported every fleeting thought of what I thought I wanted to do with myself. It was stay-at-home mom, go back to school, start my own business (or six of them), become a jewelry maker, talent manager, and a few other things, and he was confused. But he went with the flow. Thank you so much for always loving me! I never knew it was fleeting. I thought I was going to do it all until I got bored. I guess the best advice is to give to another survivor is to give the freedom and space until they can figure out what is right. A neutral listening ear can also help, in the form of a pastor, mentor, life coach, or counselor, to guide the process along. The feelings of guilt were sometimes unbearable when it came to parenting my children. I wanted them to have the best of me, and I was in an unstable state of mind. All I wanted I was to find my way around cancer and be able to figure out what was next for me. My three sons mean the world to me, and not being able to give them the structure or social time I felt they needed hurt. *I often wondered, Was I being a good enough mom? Was I too focused on me and not enough time on them?*

## Reflection:

I dislike it when people talk too much and too loudly, especially as soon as you wake up. It's annoying and everybody's breath stinks.

# IGNORANCE
# IS NOT BLISS

BREAST CANCER COMES TO take from you. It is one's own responsibility to stand up and say, "I am the boss. You are an unwelcomed foreign visitor, and you must go!" An invasion is literally taking place, and you have got to "man up or woman up" and protect your land. Your body is your land. Of course, we cannot always predict the enemy's invasion, but what we can do is act quickly and wisely once you have the knowledge that the breast cancer has invaded because early detection is key. Never waste time or allow fear to paralyze you into doing nothing. Here are a few things to consider in proactive manner in maintaining healthy habits to decrease chances of a diagnosis.

1. You must be aware of your family history. Are you predisposed?
2. Are you high risk? You need to speak candidly and freely to your health-care professionals to be assessed properly.
3. What are your lifestyle choices? Are you getting enough exercise for your particular height, weight, and age? Do you drink and smoke? Do you have a healthy diet and consume enough water?
4. Are you at a high level of stress?
5. Do you get adequate amounts of rest and relaxation, as well as sleeping hours?
6. Are you maintaining regular checkups and appointments?
7. Do you have a faith walk?

## FAMILY HISTORY

These are a few things I would recommend to consider on a day-to-day before you or anyone else you know to think upon as it relates to healthy outlook. If you know your family has a history of cancer, this is usually a good indicator to stay proactive and take preventive measures to your health, making positive choices, and being well-informed. As blessed people, sometimes we take our days for granted when we are well and do not consider that maybe, one day, things could change. I urge you to ask questions about those family members who have died. What was the cause of death? Were they healthy? If they did have cancer, what kind was it, and did it spread? It is uncommon for us to be as detailed and open about these things. But times are changing rapidly, and our health should be number one priority. Keep a journal of these things for future references and to teach the younger children as well. If there is a perpetual of health concern in an area, specifically cancer, that is more than enough information to be on guard with supporting a healthy lifestyle.

## RISK FACTORS

Risk factors can be so many things such as age, weight, family history, alcohol consumption, smoking, oral contraceptives, exposure to estrogen, radiation, diet, exercise, stress, gender, dense breasts, gene mutation, getting older, and reproductive history are a few but not at all an exhaustive list of risk factors. If you know you are high risk again, the choices you make will become healthier and wiser. The best person at doing this is nonexempt at all, but at least your chances are lower. If there is a slight notice of change, you can act fast at early detection because this is what saves lives. Unfortunately there is no bullet proof way to keep cancer away at this point in time, but we are on the brink of a cure any day now! I remain hopeful that we are closer than we have ever been in history. We must pray and advocate for proper research and to petition our government to make changes to our health-care system. We can also ask our PCP to request for genetic testing to make better decisions with health-care plans.

## LIFESTYLE

Everyone knows that drinking alcohol and smoking increases chances of disease and death. In a nut shell, we need to love our body enough not to take it into a slow death with intoxication and oppression of foreign items. You increase your chances significantly, especially if you have other risk factors to add. Life is worth living, free from any sickness and diseases! We all will leave this life one day, but it doesn't have to be because you added insult to injury by being unhealthy. I strongly encourage you to do your part and help your body to build up naturally enough to help fight any invasion.

Coffee lovers and soddie pop drinkers, you will be amazed at the wonderful effects of giving up the ingredients of the most beloved beverage choices. I speak from experience; it is not a good idea to consume these on a daily basis. I had to fight very hard not to add the caffeine to my daily intake, but it was too much sugar to consume. Most people know the physical aspects of caffeine but rarely consider the outcome and negative side effects of the drink in excess. I experienced skin problems, dehydration, false sense of energy, kidney infections, cysts, and tumors due to increase intake of sugar consumed in drinks. There are many alternatives with a healthier outcome of gaining energy or a boost. We could increase intake of water, get adequate amounts of sleep/rest, incorporate taking vitamins, get plenty of exercise, and change into a well-balanced and nutritious diet. Our bodies are made up of 60 percent of water; and in order to maintain a healthy balance, we should at least consume about two to three liters daily to maintain the average level.

## STRESS

In my opinion, I believe this is the biggest contributor not only to cancer but too many other diseases as well—if we can maintain a balance in life with home, work, and health and finance, the four major areas that contribute to stress. We could eliminate so many things. In the African American community, there are so many stigmas and myths associated with mental health counseling that it discouraged people in the urban community not to open up to be strong, to keep quiet about what's wrong, and pray about it. This has been engraved in our culture through tradition and has left a mark on how we handle stress. Stress is then bottled-up, packed, and buried, never ever unpacked, inspected, and dealt with. The pressures of life will get the best of any person and lead them to dealing with sickness and disease. If you can communicate with trusted sources about life's problems of worries, you will decrease stress levels along with maintaining a good healthy diet. A big resource in the black community is spiritual leaders, family, close friends, and maybe a network group if the person is willing to partake.

I highly recommend speaking to a neutral party which is very much easier than talking to someone who may be biased at times. There is no obligation to be perceived a certain way. Stress busters or coping skills are a good starting point to handling stress. Please consider today looking up help in your local area or other easy, accessible areas to help process life's problems.

## SLEEP

My favorite pastime is sleeping. You can cancel so many emotional and mental battles by simple addition to schedule by resting and gaining enough hours of sleep. Many of people today are facing many tasks and responsibilities that, by the time bedtime comes, it is just another thing on the list:

1. Workplace

2. Laundry
3. Shopping
4. Church
5. Bills
6. Dinner
7. Homework
8. Sleep

But we should make a conscious effort to slow down and schedule time to rest and sleep as well. What we do not finish today, we can finish tomorrow. And things get easier. Our tasks seem smaller, and we get to live another day well rested, easy going. Sleeping properly will leave you less irritable and moody. You should also consider blood pressure and heart health as well because our bodies function as one whole unit; and if one area of our being is strained, it will be a domino effect or trigger for the next thing to problematic. Sleep and rest are not the same. You can get sleep, but it may not be good restful sleep. Some things that may hinder sleep can be anxieties, worries, finances, relationships, health problems, pain, trauma, and many other things. Consult a physician always to be certain there aren't any medical reasons that sleep is being hindered. Otherwise, change the schedule and put yourself at the top of your to-do list (especially to working moms and wives). Many of us are champions to our families, but it is a disservice to function on empty day in and day out. Go to sleep.

## REGULAR DOCTOR VISITS

Be your best health advocate. I cannot preach this enough. It is better to be overchecked than to be deficient in your visits. It is a good practice to be proactive in the doctor/patient relationships. If you can get a potential problem early and make necessary adjustments, the better prognosis and perhaps the easier it is to treat any health problems. It is pretty self-explanatory. If we need to have a separate calendar specifically for follow-ups, screenings, and regular checkups, we could potentially decrease our chances of needing emergency procedures or any major problems when we notate and discuss every single change in our body with our very friendly and patient health-care team. However, if you are uncomfortable or nervous about communicating with doctors, it is advised to always take notes of questions or concerns before appointments. Take a loved one or friend and simply speak out to nurses and others involved. There may be a problem in communication areas due to feeling like your concerns or thoughts do not matter, but a good doctor truly cares about making sure their patients are educated and at peace with their health. If you are not regular with appointments, you could potentially be the very key issue in discovering something that needs attention.

If you are a good patient, these are regular practices, and your doctor does not have to worry if you will keep scheduled appointments. Continue to be educated and learn how to help your help as much as possible with your health. It is your primary responsibility to be good to you and then hold others responsible to do the same. You can always get a new team if needed but don't fire your team if you have no intentions on taking care of yourself and following recommended proceedings. There is no shame in second opinions. It is your body, your health, your future, your own perceptions. By all means, if you have unnecessary stress about seeing your doctors, please communicate this topic of being regular which can be the difference between life and death in some cases.

Many have heard if you had waited any longer before coming in, you would have had a heart attack, went into a coma, had a stroke, or even died. In the day we are now living in, there is no excuse not to do your best to take your health serious enough to consult with a health-care team to make sure you are well. Here are some of the signs of the importance of the last stated session (be regular with doctor visits). If you notice anything new in your body, mood, appetite, hair, nails, moles, facial hair, pain, aches, weight changes, rashes, lumps, nodules, consistent coughs or colds, even dental and eye changes, notify a medical-care team and seek help. Our bodies speak to us every time something is going on; but we mostly ignore, dismiss, or not pay attention until the signs and symptoms worsen. In this case, treatments and prognosis can be most difficult or not as effective as it would if we would react at the first signs of disease. One of the most important things we learn is that early detection saves lives. The sooner you find the problem, the higher the chances of survival. I agree that this statement is true, but a better way to view "saving lives" is to understand no detection saves lives. Not receiving a terminal diagnosis is what truly saves lives, as it relates to breast health.

# FAITH WALK

> Be strong and courageous, do not be afraid
> or tremble in dread before them, for it is the Lord
> your God who goes with you. He will not fail
> you or abandon you. (Deuteronomy 31:6)

I AM NOT SURE HOW people of no faith are able to come through some of life's hardest times without a personal walk with a Savior. In the event you get a bad report or negative results, having a strong faith walk will help diminish doubt, fear, and cause you to reflect upon the good things only or focus on the promises rather than the problem. It will also help your emotions stabilize, and the results will more than likely come back positive due to the seeds of hope and faith already stored up. I'm not sure what my current state of mind or health would be if I did not have a solid faith in God. Perhaps if I was not able to stand on the Word, I may not even be living today. Some people live many years after tragedies, trials, and tribulations and still not acknowledge the power of God's grace and mercy.

> Now faith is the assurance [title deed, con-
> firmation] of things hoped for [divinely guaran-
> teed], and the evidence of things not seen [the
> conviction of their reality—faith comprehends as
> fact what cannot be experienced by the physical
> senses]. (Hebrews 11:1)

In the event that you cannot see what you hope for or aspire to have, you can reach for the expectation that you hold in your heart. I was unable to grasp the truth of the Word in the beginning of my personal journey, but I was not willing to give up. I desired to live so I hung on every word, even while in pain, while I cried, after every visit to the doctor. I am no better than anyone else, and I recognized how undeserving I was to benefit from having another chance to be better and do better. True faith happened when I could not trace anything in the natural, yet I made a decision to go against the grain with my thoughts and actions to move forward in my belief that I would live.

> For it is by grace [God's remarkable compassion and favor drawing you to Christ] that you have been saved [actually delivered from judgment and given eternal life] through faith. And this [salvation] is not of yourselves [not through your own effort], but it is the underserved, gracious] gift of God. (Ephesians 2:8)

God freely gives us all the gift of salvation if we will believe. The drawing that happens to bring us out of the old dark ways of living into a new and righteous living is his grace. We cannot earn it by law or works or deeds. When judgment could have gone forth against us, the Lord decides to extend his hand of mercy. Our efforts are absolutely flawed and simply not enough to be saved. It may not be cancer or any other illness; but if you want to know him for real, seek him!

> And we know [with great confidence] that God [who I deeply concerned about us] causes all things to work together [as a plan] for good for those who love God, to those who are called according to His plan and purpose.—Romans 8:28

There is a perfect purpose for every pain we go through. Even when it looked like things are all messed up and going wrong, we cannot lose. Somehow everything will work out fine. Do not panic. He cares for us all.

> Be assured that the testing of your faith [through experience] produces endurance [leading to spiritual maturity, and inner peace]. (James 1:3)

Life will teach you a thing or two. It shows me every day the level of maturity can always be stretched. At the reoccurrence, I can honestly say the Lord had built within me a true assurance that he was the truth and that his Word was good. I had to make a decision. Could I believe Him when He said I was healed? The spirit of the Lord spoke within me and said, "I did not change my mind. You are healed!" God does not make any mistakes. He is not schizophrenic, and he is not a liar! Try living in this mind-set and see inner peace will flood you, and growth happens. Sometimes I don't recognize my own self.

> Keeping your faith [leaning completely on God with absolute trust and confidence in His guidance] and having a good conscience; for some [people] have rejected [their moral compass] and have made a shipwreck of their faith. (1 Timothy 1:19)

There is no time for room and space for anything else other than God alone. He needs no help. His grace is sufficient. We are not to forget the foundation of our belief; otherwise, it will not end well. If we are not careful to stand on the truth of the Word, we will not make a victorious end. Now that you have gotten a good idea of some things to consider before allowing anything to conquer you be it sickness or any other issue, perhaps this will get you on a good start or maybe hit the restart button of your life to focus more on the

Word. I wished I had good practices of these things prior to being diagnosed. It may not always change the course, but it would definitely help in the process. I'm only one survivor of millions around the world. I can only share with you from my viewpoint and taken in some advice from great health-care professionals. I will continue to work on being health conscious. It is a good feeling just thinking of better living skills that produce longevity and productivity.

# GLOSSARY

## (Not an Exhaustive List)

*Aggressive* (uh-GREH-siv): In medicine, describes a tumor or disease that forms, grows, or spreads quickly. It may also describe treatment that is more severe or intense than usual.

*Alopecia* (A-loh-PEE-shuh): The lack or loss of hair from areas of the body where hair is usually found. Alopecia can be a side effect of some cancer treatments.

*Axillary lymph node* (AK-sih-LAYR-ee limf node): A lymph node in the armpit region that drains lymph from the breast and nearby areas.

*Benign* (beh-NINE): Not cancerous. Benign tumors may grow larger but do not spread to other parts of the body. Also called nonmalignant.

*Biopsy* (BY-op-see): The removal of cells or tissues for examination by a pathologist. The pathologist may study the tissue under a microscope or perform other tests on the cells or tissue. There are many different types of biopsy procedures. The most common types include: (1) incisional biopsy in which only a sample of tissue is removed; (2) excisional biopsy in which an entire lump or suspicious area is removed; and (3) needle biopsy in which a sample of tissue or fluid is removed with a needle. When a wide needle is used, the procedure is called a core biopsy. When a thin needle is used, the procedure is called a fine-needle aspiration biopsy.

*Breast cancer* (brest KAN-ser): Cancer that forms in tissues of the breast. The most common type of breast cancer is ductal carcinoma, which begins in the lining of the milk ducts (thin tubes that carry milk from the lobules of the breast to the nipple). Another type of breast cancer is lobular carcinoma, which begins in the lobules (milk glands) of the breast. Invasive breast cancer is breast cancer that has spread from where it began in the breast ducts or lobules to surrounding normal tissue. Breast cancer occurs in both men and women although male breast cancer is rare.

*Breast reconstruction* (brest REE-kun-STRUK-shun): Surgery to rebuild the shape of the breast after a mastectomy.

*Carcinoma* (KAR-sih-NOH-muh): Cancer that begins in the skin or in tissues that line or cover internal organs.

*Carcinoma in situ* (KAR-sih-NOH-muh in SY-too): A group of abnormal cells that remain in the place where they first formed. They have not spread. These abnormal cells may become cancer and spread into nearby normal tissue. Also called stage 0 disease.

*Chemotherapy* (KEE-moh-THAYR-uh-pee): Treatment that uses drugs to stop the growth of cancer cells, either by killing the cells or by stopping them from dividing. Chemotherapy may be given by mouth, injection, or infusion, or on the skin, depending on the type and stage of the cancer being treated. It may be given alone or with other treatments, such as surgery, radiation therapy, or biologic therapy.

*Core needle biopsy* (…NEE-dul BY-op-see): The removal of a tissue sample with a wide needle for examination under a microscope. Also called core biopsy.

*Cyst* (sist): A closed, saclike pocket of tissue that can form anywhere in the body. It may be filled with fluid, air, pus, or other material. Most cysts are benign (not cancer).

*DCIS*: A noninvasive condition in which abnormal cells are found in the lining of a breast duct. The abnormal cells have not spread outside the duct to other tissues in the breast. In some cases, DCIS may become invasive cancer and spread to other tissues. At this time, there is no way to know which lesions could become invasive. Also called ductal carcinoma in situ and intraductal carcinoma.

*Ductal carcinoma* (DUK-tul KAR-sih-NOH-muh): The most common type of breast cancer. It begins in the lining of the milk ducts (thin tubes that carry milk from the lobules of the breast to the nipple). Ductal carcinoma may be either ductal carcinoma in situ (DCIS) or invasive ductal carcinoma. DCIS is a noninvasive condition in which abnormal cells are found in the lining of a breast duct and have not spread outside the duct to other tissues in the breast. In some cases, DCIS may become invasive cancer. In invasive ductal carcinoma, cancer has spread outside the breast duct to surrounding normal tissue. It can also spread through the blood and lymph systems to other parts of the body.

*HER2 negative* (...NEH-guh-tiv): Describes cancer cells that do not have a large amount of a protein called HER2 on their surface. In normal cells, HER2 helps to control cell growth. Cancer cells that are HER2 negative may grow more slowly and are less likely to recur (come back) or spread to other parts of the body than cancer cells that have a large amount of HER2 on their surface. Checking for the amount of HER2 on some types of cancer cells may help plan treatment. These cancers include breast, bladder, ovarian, pancreatic, and stomach cancers. Also called human epidermal growth factor receptor 2 negative.

*HER2-positive cancer* (...PAH-zih-tiv KAN-ser): Describes cancer cells that have too much of a protein called HER2 on their surface. In normal cells, HER2 helps control cell growth. When it is made in larger than normal amounts by cancer cells, the cells may grow more quickly and are more likely to spread to other parts of the body. Checking to see if a cancer is HER2 positive may help plan treatment, which may include drugs that kill HER2-positive cancer cells. Cancers that may be HER2 positive include breast, bladder, pancreatic, ovarian, and stomach cancers. Also called c-erbB-2-positive cancer and human epidermal growth factor receptor 2-positive cancer.

*Invasive breast cancer* (in-VAY-siv brest KAN-ser): Cancer that has spread from where it began in the breast to surrounding normal tissue. The most common type of invasive breast cancer is invasive ductal carcinoma, which begins in the lining of the milk ducts (thin tubes that carry milk from the lobules of the breast to the nipple). Another type is invasive lobular carcinoma, which begins in the lobules (milk glands) of the breast. Invasive breast cancer can spread through the blood and lymph systems to other parts of the body. Also called infiltrating breast cancer.

*Localized* (LOH-kuh-lized): In medicine, describes disease that is limited to a certain part of the body. For example, localized cancer is usually found only in the tissue or organ where it began and has not spread to nearby lymph nodes or to other parts of the body. Some localized cancers can be completely removed by surgery.

*Lumpectomy* (lum-PEK-toh-mee): An operation to remove the cancer and some normal tissue around it, but not the breast itself. Some lymph nodes under the arm may be removed for biopsy. Part of the chest wall lining may also be removed if the cancer is near it. Also called breast-conserving surgery, breast-sparing surgery, partial mastectomy, quadrantectomy, and segmental mastectomy.

*Lymph node* (limf node): A small bean-shaped structure that is part of the body's immune system. Lymph nodes filter substances that travel through the lymphatic fluid, and they contain lymphocytes (white blood cells) that help the body fight infection and disease. There are hundreds of lymph nodes found throughout the body. They are connected to one another by lymph vessels. Clusters of lymph nodes are found in the neck, axilla (underarm), chest, abdomen, and groin. For example, there are about twenty to forty lymph nodes in the axilla. Also called lymph gland.

*Lymphedema* (LIM-fuh-DEE-muh): A condition in which extra lymph fluid builds up in tissues and causes swelling. It may occur in an arm or leg if lymph vessels are blocked, damaged, or removed by surgery.

*Malignant* (muh-LIG-nunt): Cancerous. Malignant cells can invade and destroy nearby tissue and spread to other parts of the body.

*Mammogram* (MA-muh-gram): An X-ray of the breast.

*Mastectomy* (ma-STEK-toh-mee): Surgery to remove part or all of the breast. There are different types of mastectomy that differ in the amount of tissue and lymph nodes removed.

*Palliative care* (PA-lee-uh-tiv kayr): Care given to improve the quality of life of patients who have a serious or life-threatening disease. The goal of palliative care is to prevent or treat as early as possible the symptoms of a disease, side effects caused by treatment of a disease, and psychological, social, and spiritual problems related to a disease or its treatment. Also called comfort care, supportive care, and symptom management.

*Prognosis* (prog-NO-sis): The likely outcome or course of a disease; the chance of recovery or recurrence.

*Radiation therapy* (RAY-dee-AY-shun THAYR-uh-pee): The use of high-energy radiation from X-rays, gamma rays, neutrons, protons, and other sources to kill cancer cells and shrink tumors. Radiation may come from a machine outside the body (external-beam radiation therapy), or it may come from radioactive material placed in the body near cancer cells (internal radiation therapy or brachytherapy). Systemic radiation therapy uses a radioactive substance, such as a radiolabeled monoclonal antibody, that travels in the blood to tissues throughout the body. Also called irradiation and radiotherapy.

*Recurrence* (ree-KER-ents): Cancer that has recurred (come back), usually after a period during which the cancer could not be detected. The cancer may come back to the same place as the original (primary) tumor or to another place in the body. Also called recurrent cancer.

*Remission* (reh-MIH-shun): A decrease in or disappearance of signs and symptoms of cancer. In partial remission, some, but not all, signs and symptoms of cancer have disappeared. In complete remission, all signs and symptoms of cancer have disappeared, although cancer still may be in the body.

*Sarcoma* (sar-KOH-muh): A type of cancer that begins in bone or in the soft tissues of the body, including cartilage, fat, muscle, blood vessels, fibrous tissue, or other connective or supportive tissue. Different types of sarcoma are based on where the cancer forms. For example, osteosarcoma forms in bone, liposarcoma forms in fat, and rhabdomyosarcoma forms in muscle. Treatment and prognosis depend on the type and grade of the cancer (how abnormal the cancer cells look under a microscope and how quickly the cancer is likely to grow and spread). Sarcoma occurs in both adults and children.

Reference: *National Cancer Institute.* NCI Dictionary of Cancer Terms.2015. Available at https://www.cancer.gov/publications/dictionaries/cancer-terms.Accessed 2/26/2020

# REFLECTIONS

AND THE LORD ANSWERED me, and said, write the vision, and make it plain upon tables, that he may run that readeth it.

> For the vision is yet for an appointed time,
> but at the end it shall speak, and not lie: though
> it tarry, wait for it; because it will surely come, it
> will not tarry. (Habakkuk 2:2–3)

It is very encouraging and healing to write daily however big or small. I encourage you in your journey in dealing with life's ups and downs to take notes and record the process. Perspective is much clearer when you can see your thoughts and your emotions written down. This process should be as natural as possible even if it's a few weeks in between entries; but I recommend trying to write weekly, if not daily. Be intentional and see the beauty unfold.

Questions to answer:

- Did you learn anything new? If so, what exactly did you learn? What were your thoughts prior to learning? These questions and those listed below are some simple writing prompts that can help you stir your journaling process and perhaps your very own book.
- How did this personal journey make you feel about your own story?

- What are some ways that you can think of that you can help someone else deal with their hardships in life?
- What are some things you do to deal with your life's trials?
- If you had the ability to change your life right now, how would your life look?
- Have you ever been misunderstood about anything? Explain how. What did that feel like?
- What is your current mood?
- When are you most powerful/or less fearful?
- Explain what are you are you fearful of. Explain why.
- How would you describe an ideal day or a good day for you?
- What does it mean to be successful?
- Do you know good tools for you to cope with stress? If so, list at least five things.

# JOURNAL

Date:

Time:

Topic:

# ABOUT THE AUTHOR

SHARON REJISTRE IS A two-time breast cancer survivor, certified life coach, and mentor. She is passionate about breast cancer awareness and educating anyone who's willing and learn to do something about the complexities of cancer. She detailed her fight with cancer in her debut book, a health autobiography entitled *Steadfast*. She currently serves as a member of Living Beyond Breast Cancer, Young Women's Initiative program, speaking and sharing her story as an advocate.

In 2014, she received the Dr. Josetta Wilkins Awards for her nonprofit Pink Orchid Cancer Foundation. She has received several certificates and awards as a speaker/presenter in seminars and conferences. She has petitioned to congress through Breast Cancer Action for continuation of funding to various federal programs. She travels throughout the states to year around to share her story and inspire others. She has been a featured speaker on the *Let's Talk About It* video series. She was featured in the 2011 publication *Getting Connected* booklet for the newly diagnosed.

Sharon holds a Bachelor of Science in psychology and a minor in criminal justice from the University of Arkansas at Pine Bluff. She resides in Hot Springs Village, AR, with her husband, Dr. Alexander Rejistre Sr., and three sons, Alex Jr., Aaron, and Anais. She enjoys family time, writing, traveling, spas, and skydiving. Her hope is to continue to reach out to underserved communities across the world, educating others to be interactive with and proactive about their health.

For more information visit: www.sharonrejistre.com